What to Eat
&
What Not to Eat

What to Eat & What not to Eat

DR. L. C. GUPTA M.D.
DR ABHISHEK GUPTA M.D

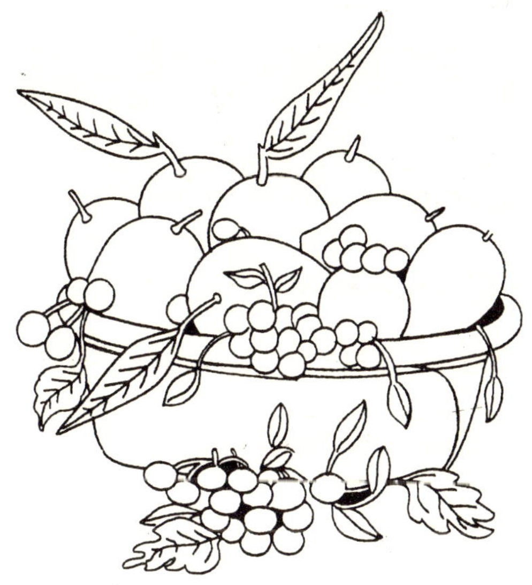

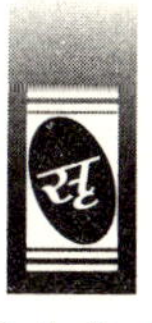

Srishti
PUBLISHERS & DISTRIBUTORS

Srishti Publishers & Distributors
N-16, C. R. Park
New Delhi 110 019
srishtipublishers@gmail.com

First published by
Srishti Publishers & Distributors in 2004
2nd impression 2012

Typeset in AGaramond 11pt. by Suresh Kumar Sharma at Srishti

Cover Design: Shivani Babbar

Printed and bound in India

Dedicated
to
Devoted
Mr. Vijay Goel
Mr. Ram Das Agarwal
Mr. Pradeep Mittal
&
Babu Ram Gupta
Fighting for the cause of
"Vaishya-unity"

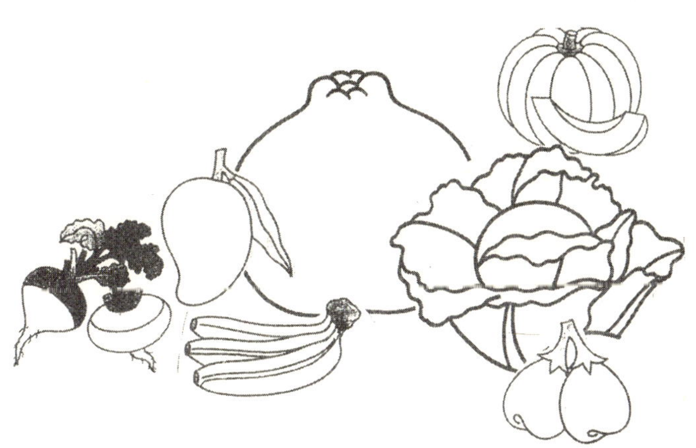

Contents

Preface

All living things need food. But every culture has its own dietary patterns based on the use of various sources of food. Some cultures may not be finding necessary to have non-vegetarian food while others are crazy for it. Although the food patterns have ensured survival, the existing pattern is not necessarily the best. Modern youth is far away from nature and has acquired artificial taste for food which is neither essential nor conducive. Present day fast food contains a greater proportion of sugar and fats resulting in malnutrition. About 3 million children are blind because of failure to choose the right kind of green vegetables in our country.

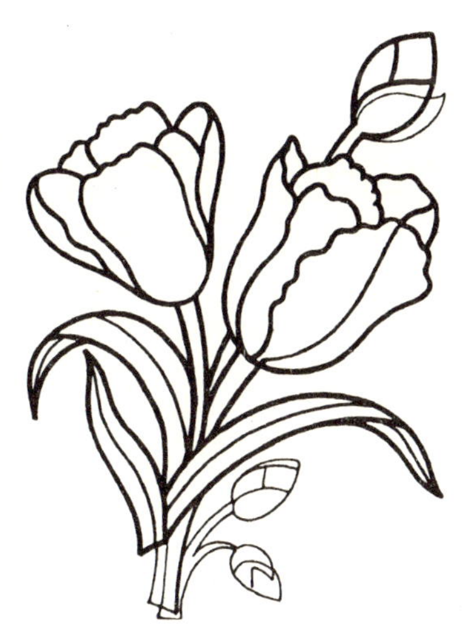

This book in the form of questions and answers is an attempt to communicate to a lay man as well as students of nutrition to what to eat and what not to eat and why so. Special attempts have been made to formulate diets for special age groups, pregnancy and sportsmen. It clears doubts and confusion of food faddism. Food values at last increases the value of book.

We are thankful to Acupressure specialist Dr. A. K. Saxena and Guptaji of Need Book Depo for their valued help.

L. C Gupta

Abhishek Gupta

Introduction

How human diet can be classified?

It can be broadly classified into two categories

(i) Vegetarian

(ii) Non Vegetarian

Does Vegetarian diet can be further classified?

Yes,

Frutarian – Consumes fruits only

Vegan – Cereals only. They don't take even milk

Lacto Vegetarian – Consume vegetables,

Lacto-ovo-vegetarian – They consume vegetables, cereals, milk and eggs.

The term 'vegetarian' used in India generally refers to lacto-vegetarian.

What about the biological aspects of vegetarianism?

Anatomically man has body structure which is akin to the vegetarian species and different from meat eating species.

Meat eating animals have sharp, pointed teeth and claws with hard pointed nails which help them in tearing easy prey while vegetarian animals have nails and claws to pluck fruits.

Carnivorus (meat eating) animals swallow their food without mastication. Their jaw moves upwards and downwards only, while herbivorus (vegetarian) animals first chew the food and then swallow, so their jaw moves in all direction i.e. left and right also.

The tongue of meat eating animals is very smooth.

Is there any change in digestive system of two animals?

The length of intestines of carnivorus animals is comparatively smaller i.e. almost equal to their body length because they have to excrete the digested flesh before it further putrefies. Man has very long intestine which cannot quickly expel the fleshy food.

The content of hydrochloric acid in gastric juice in vegetarian species in much less and so they are unable to digest meat easily. Saliva of flesh water is acidic while that of vegetarians is alkaline.

The liver and kidney of meat eater are larger in proportion to enable them to secrete larger amounts of hepatic juices and excrete the waste products, while that of vegetarians is purposely smaller in size.

What is the visual impression of different foods?

Visually no human beings feel disgusted at the sight or smell or fruits, vegetables or cereals while many people have a repulsive

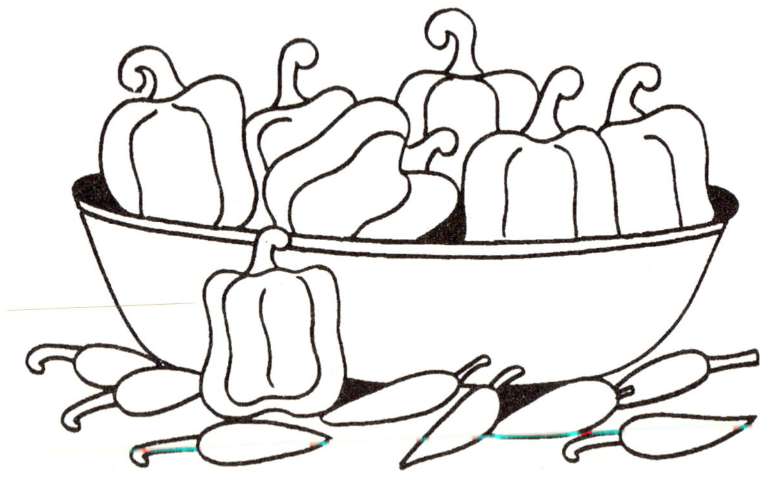

Proteins

What do you understand by proteins?

The word protein means necessary for life because vital parts of nucleus are protein in nature. The term protein means 'to take first place' and was introduced by Dutch chemist Mulder in 1838.

How much proteins body contains?

Protein is a constituent of every living cell. Half of the dry weight and 20% of total weight of body is protein. 50% of it is in muscles. 10% in skin, 20% in bone and cartilage and rest in other tissues and fluids. Urine and bile does not contain protein.

What is the chemical composition of proteins?

These are complex substances made up of many aminoacids. Amino acids are basic units from which protein is synthesized and into which it is converted in the course of digestion. Protein molecules are much large with a molecular weight of 40 million compared to 180 for glucose.

Chemically what are aminoacids?

Aminoacids are composed of carboxyl group (COOH), a hydrogen atom (H) an amino group (NH2) and an amino acid radical attached to a carbon atom.

```
COOH
   \
H → C — R
   /
NH2
```

How many types of amino acids are available?

There are twenty different naturally occuring aminoacids are there. Out of which 8 are essential required for childs growth

Isolucine

Leucine

Lysine

Methionine

Phenylalanine

Threonine

Tryptophan

Valine & Histidine

What about nitrogen group of amino acids?

Nitrogen is not found in carbohydrate and fats. On an average milk contains 15% nitrogen, meat 16% and cereals 17%.

How to classify aminoacid?

Functionally aminoacids, are classified into

(i) Essential (indispensable)

(ii) Non essential (dispensable)

Indispensable aminoacid is that which cannot be synthesized by body, sufficient to meet the needs for growth and maintenance.

What are endogenous and exogenous proteins?

Endogenous proteins are derived from body tissues and is reflected in the excretion of nitrogen containing substance creatinine. It is an indication of basal energy expenditure.

Exogenous proteins are proteins from dietary sources outside the body. It results in excretion of urea which fluctuates with dietary intake.

What about food as a source of aminoacids?

Nutritive value of food protein lies in aminoacid composition. Some food such as gelatin contains only one protein while meat contains hemoglobin, myoglobin, elastin and collagen. Milk contains casein and lactolbumin and glutenin are found in wheat.

Can one aminoacid be changed into another?

Yes, Methionine an essential aminoacid can be converted to cystine, but cystine cannot be converted to methionine. Similarly phenylalanine can be converted to tyrosine but not vice versa. Thus cystine and tyrosine are sometimes classified as semi essential aminoacids.

What is limiting aminoacid?

The aminoacid present in smallest amount than required is known as limiting amino acid. Lysine is limiting aminoacid of wheat while methionine is of pulses.

What are the common abnormalities in aminoacid metabolism?

Some infants are not able to produce enzyme necessary for phenylalanine metabolism. Accumulated phenylalanine has adverse effect on nervous system. Child may be mentally retarded.

Homocystinuria is failure to convert cystine to methionine is second most inborn error of metabolism. It is caused by lack of vitamin B_6.

Is supplementation of aminoacid possible?

Why not? Lysine is an limiting aminoacid of wheat, to compensate lysine is being added while making 'modern bread.'

How are proteins classified?

These may be classified in many ways

1. Simple protein
   Conjugated protein
2. Derived complete proteins
   Partially complete
   Incomplete
3. Class I proteins
   Class II proteins

What are simple proteins?

These on hydrolysis by acid and alkalies or enzymes yield only aminoacids or their derivatives. Albumin and globulins are example of it and are within all body cells and in blood serum. These are found in keratin, collagen and elastin in supportive tissues of the body such as hair and nails, globin in hemoglobin and myoglobin, glutenin in wheat, legumin in peas and lacto albumin and lacto globulin in milk.

What are conjugated proteins?

These are simple proteins combined with non protein substance. It includes lipoproteins vehicle to transport fats in blood. Nucleoproteins are the proteins of cell nuclei. Phosphoproteins such as casein is found in milk and ovovitellin in eggs.

How we get derived proteins?

There are substances resulting from the decomposition of simple and conjugated proteins.

What do you understand by complete proteins?

Proteins containing all essential aminoacids in proportion to maintain proper growth are described as complete proteins, high biological value protein. They contain 33% essential and 60% non essential aminoacids. All animal proteins except gelatin which

What do you understand by limiting aminoacids?

The aminoacid present in smaller amount than required is called limiting aminoacid. Arginine is the limiting aminoacid in casein as is methionine in fish and eggs. Cereals lack in lysine and legumes in methionine. Both soya and nuts contain some of all essential aminoacids but are sufficiently limited in one or more making these less effective than animal proteins.

Can proteins be supplemented?

Yes it is possible to simulate a complete protein by supplying two vegetable proteins that complement each other. For example wheat lacking in lysine when taken with pulses which are lacking in methionine will provide a mixture containing all aminoacids. On the same line small amount of milk with wheat or rice will provide missing aminoacid and will enhance the biological value of proteins of cereals.

How to extend high quality protein?

The essential aminoacids are present in animal proteins in such a way that small quantities of animal products will make up the essential aminoacid deficits of plant proteins. Example of protein extension are chicken and rice, macroni with cheese and cereals with milk.

Are concentrated source of plant proteins useful?

It is wise to rely on more concentrated source of plant proteins such as dried beans, peas or noodles

What are the functions of proteins?

(i) Sources of calories – Proteins are potential source of energy. Each gram of protein gives 4.1 calories.

(ii) Maintenance of growth – Proteins constitute the chief solid matter of muscles, organs and endocrine glands. Matrix of bones, teeth, nails, hair every living cell has protein. First need of aminoacid is to supply material for building and continuous replacement of cell proteins throughout life.

(iii) Regulation of body process – Proteins have some highly specialised functions in regulation of body processes.

- Contractile proteins, myosin and actin regulate muscle contraction.
- Catalytic proteins are enzymes to facilitate each step of digestion, absorption and anabolism.
- Nucleoproteins contain the blue print for the synthesis of all body proteins.
- Hornomal proteins control metabolic processes.
- Immune proteins maintain the body's resistance against infection.
- Blood proteins – Hemoglobin is involved in transport of oxygen and carbon dioxide and maintains acid base balance.

How proteins are digested?

Total protein requiring digestion may be 150 gm or so, about 90 gram from food and 60 gram from an endogenous source. Within the digestive tract endogenous and exogenous are treated at par.

The saliva contains no proteslytic enzyme and thus the only action in the month is an increase in surface area of food mass as a result of chewing. Most of the hydrolysis occurs in stomach and duodenum. There protein molecules are broken in smaller fragments. Enzymes are recreated in their inactive form and are activated when their need is for protein hydrolysis. Each enzyme is highly specific, and hydrolysis only one type of protein. The rate of digestion depends on rate of absorption.

What are the important enzymes used in protein digestion?

Enzyme and Location	Action
<u>Stomach</u>	
Pepsinogen	Activated to pepsin by HCL splits
Pepsin	peptide chain where tyrosin furnishes amino group
<u>Small intestine</u>	
Trypsinogen	Activated to trypsin by enterokinase
Trypsin	Splits peptide chain where lysine or arginine furnishes carboxyl group
Chymotrypsinogen	Activated to chymotrypsin by trypsin
Chymotrypsin	Splits peptide chain where tryptophane, methionine, tryosine provides carboxyl group.
<u>Intestinal Nucosa</u>	
Aminopeptidase	Splits peptide linkage to terminal group
Carboxypeptidase	Splits peptide linkage next to terminal carboxyl group.

Where most of digestion of protein occurs?

Digestion occurs in upper half of intestine. In lower half these same protein splitting enzymes digest 50-70% of endogenous proteins resulting from loss of intestinal cells.

What do you understand by coefficient of digestibility?

The digestibility of protein is the percentage of protein intake that is available for absorption.

Calculation is

$$CD = \frac{\text{N Intake} - (\text{N - fecal N on protein free diet})}{\text{N intake}} \times 100$$

Milk and eggs have digestibility co-efficient of about 97, meat, fish, poultry less than that and plant proteins 75-80%.

The digestibility can often be improved if foods have been heated with strong acid/alkalies.

What is the effect of protein dematuration?

Proteolytic enzymes not only bring about the splitting of peptide linkage but they also splits the cross links. During moderate heating some of these cross linkages are broken and it facilitates digestion. But in certain cases excessive heating results in formation of linkages that are resistant to the digestive enzyme. As a result aminoacids don't become available to body.

How enzyme inhibitors act?

Some foods such as beans and soya bean contains substances that inhibit the activity of enzyme such as trypsin. Heating inactivates these inhibitors thereby improving the digestibility of protein.

How absorption of protein occurs?

About 12% of free aminoacids are absorbed in stomach, 60% in small intestine and 28% in colon. Aminoacids are absorbed in portal circulation. Rate of absorption is dependent upon.

- Total load of aminoacids released through digestion

- Proportions of various aminoacid present in mixture.
- Uptake of aminoacids by tissues.
- Availability of carriers to the aminoacids into mucosal cells.

What about the metabolism of proteins?

Absorbed aminoacids are released from intestinal wall into portal vein and carried to liver. If aminoacids are not needed they will be excreted as urea in urine. Some are synthesized into plasma proteins by liver and rest are released in blood circulation. From blood aminoacids are taken up by individual cells using them in synthesis of a specific protein. For this all aminoacids are required at a time. If they are not available cells will release aminoacids to be taken up by another cells or used for energy.

Does sufficient calories are needed for protein synthesis?

For protein synthesis to proceed at an optimum rate the calorie intake must be sufficient to supply the energy needs. A deficiency of calories forces the use of some dietary and tissue proteins for energy.

What is nitrogen equilibrium?

It is the state of balance where nitrogen intake is equal to nitrogen excreted.

What is positive nitrogen balance?

It is the state in which intake of nitrogen exceeds the excretion. It shows that new protein tissues are formed as in growing stage of child or during pregnancy or in athletic training. But there is no over storage of proteins.

What is negative nitrogen balance?

In this excretion of nitrogen exceeds the intake. It means person is loosing nitrogen from tissues more rapidly than it is being replaced.

(i) the quality of protein is poor

(ii) the amount feed is inadequate for tissue replacement

(iii) calorie content of diet is inadequate so tissues are being broken to supply energy

(iv) injury, fever/diseases causing excessive break down of tissues.

What is the daily requirement of proteins?

Daily requirement of protein is 1 gm per kilogram of body weight Table showing daily protein requirement.

Age	Requirement
Man 60 Kg	60 gram
Woman 45 Kg	45 gram
Later half pregnancy	55 gram
Lactation	65 gram
Children	
Up to 1 year	10-13 grams
Up to 2 years	15 grams
Up to 4 years	20 gram
5 to 9 years	28-33 gram
10 to 12 years	40 gram
13 to 16 years	45-55 gram

On what factors the proteins requirements depends?

- Essential aminoacids must be present in sufficient amount to meet needs to tissue regeneration.

- Diet should yield sufficient calories.
- Growth needs of infants and children increases the protein requirement per Kg of body weight.
- Development of maternal tissue and fetus increases protein requirement.
- Fever/disease/T.B. needs additional protein for repletion.
- Emotional stress increases protein catabolism.
- Sufficient proteins for adults is needed to cover daily nitrogen losses in urine/feces, desquamated skin, hair, perspiration etc.

What is the requirement of essential aminoacids?

Aminoacid requirement per Kg/ body weight mg/day

Aminoacid	4-6 Month	10-12 years	Adults
Histidine	33	–	–
Isoleucine	83	28	12
Leucine	135	42	16
Lysine	99	44	12
Methionine and cystine	49	22	10
Phenylamine and tyrosine	141	22	16
Threonine	68	28	8
Tryptophane	21	4	3
Valima	92	25	14

On a weight basis infants requirements are several times higher, because of high rate of tissue synthesis during infancy. For adults only 20% of total nitrogen should be supplied by essential aminoacids. While for infants it goes up to 35%.

What are the important sources of proteins?

Important sources of proteins gm/100 gram.

Food	Protein	Food	Protein
Wheat	11.8	Egg Hen	13.3
Rice	7.0	Fish	21
Maize	11.1	Mutton	18.5
Bengal gram	17.1	Milk	3.5
Moong dal	24.0	Ground nut	26.7
Masoor	25.1	Milk human	1.2
Soya bean	42.0		

In India instead of protein deficiency there is deficiency of calories, because stable diet consists of wheat/rice and dal giving sufficient amount of proteins.

Animal proteins are costlier and is not a must.

What will happen if proteins are consumed liberally?

Consumption of a high protein diet is wasteful, however, since the body does not store protein as such. Excess aminoacids are deaminized and metabolized as fats and carbohydrate. Protein foods entail more work for liver and kidneys.

What are other side effects of consumption of high proteins?

High proteins may prove undesirable. As consumption of protein increases calcium absorption is reduced.

With an increased in nitrogenous waste more water is required to excrete them. Premature and young infants are not able to excrete additional nitrogen.

Persons who have renal failure also cannot excrete large amount of wastes and blood urea levels are elevated.

Animal proteins are also source of large amount of saturated fats and carbohydrates.

What will happen in case of protein deficiency?

Children suffer most due to parents ignorance or abuse. Protein intake which fails to meet the requirement leads first to depletion of tissue reserves and then to a lowering of blood protein levels. Nutritional oedema is a chemical sign. Protein deficiency sometimes becomes abruptly evidence when an infection, injury or surgery do take place.

What do you understand by malnutrition?

It may be due to improper or inadequate food intake or may result from inadequate absorption of food. Deficient supply of food, poverty, food, faddism all may cause it. Certain abnormalities of metabolism may also cause it.

What do you understand by marasmus?

Clinical picture is of general starvation. It may be due to primarily of inadequate calories and protein deficiency.

There will be failure of gaining weight. Skin becomes wrinkled due to loss of subcutaneous fat. Face looks like of a monkey. Abdomen may be distended. There may be associated vitamin deficiency.

When you will say that child is suffering from Kwashiorkor?

It is a basically deficiency of protein followed by lack of calories. Protein is the most limiting nutrient clinical features include –

- Failure to grow in both weight and length. There will be weak, thin and wasted muscles.

- Child will be irritative.
- There will be accumulation of fluid in tissues causing them to be soft and spongy especially in lower limbs.
- Skin crusts, dry and may form ulcers.
- Hair becomes sparse, brown loosing its pigmentation.
- Loss of appetite, vomiting and diarrhea.
- Liver may enlarge
- Child may develop anemia.

Most important serum albumin level. Indian old food 'Sattu' is very helpful being mixture of gur + wheat + chana.

How will you differentiate between marasmus and kwashiorkor?

Table showing difference between marasmus and kwashiorkor.

Feature	Marasmus	Kwashiorkor
Primary cause	Deficiency of calories	Deficiency of proteins
Wasting	Thin, lean and skinny	Less obvious, child looks flabby; Moon face
Muscle wasting	Severe	Sometimes lees
Loss of weight	marked	Marked by edema
Appetite	Usually good	Poor
Skin changes	None	Depigmented
Hair change	Slight	Often sparse
Liver	Not enlarged	Enlarged
Diarrhoea	Not necessary	Present

Fats

Fats are most concentrated source of calories. They are valued for the enhancement of food palatability.

What is the composition of fats?

Lipids include fats, oils and fat like substances. It has greasy feel which is insoluble in water but soluble in ether, alcohol and benzene. These are composed of three elements. Like carbohydrate it is composed of three elements carbon, hydrogen and ozygen. It differs from carbohydrate that the ratio of oxygen to carbon and hydrogen is much lower 1:2 in simple carbohydrates and 1:30 in simple fats. Lower amount of oxygen makes it more concentrated source of energy.

What are fatty acids?

The main constituents of all lipids are fatty acids. They consist of chain of CO_2 atoms with a methyl group at one end and carboxyl COOH group at other end.

What type of fatty acids are available?

Fatty acids are 'saturated' or unsaturated. A fatty acid in which each of carbon atoms in chain has two hydrogen atoms attached to it is saturated. An unsaturated fatty acid is one in which a hydrogen atom is missing from each of two adjoining carbon atoms.

How lipids are classified?

These are classified into 3 (i) simple lipids (ii) compound lipids and (iii) derived lipids.

- Simple lipids are esters of glycerol and fatty acids.

Monoglyceroids are formed by combining a fatty acid with one of hydroxyl group of glycerol molecule. Diglyceride contain two fatty acids and tringlyceride also referred to as neutral fats containing three fatty acids.

- Compound lipids – There are esters of glycerol and fatty acids with substitution of other components such as carbohydrate phosphate or nitrogenous groupings.
- Derived lipids – These include fatty acids, alcohols, glycerols and sterols, carotenoids and fat soluble vitamins A,D,E and K.

What do you understand by P/S ratio?

The proportion of unsaturated to saturated fatty acid in a fat is expressed as P/S ratio. Higher the ratio the higher is the proportion of unsaturated fatty acid and more likely it is a liquid.

What are the characteristic of fats?

The nature of fats, their hardness melting point and flavour is determined by the length of carbon chain and level of saturation of fatty acids. Pure tringlycerides are tasteless, they have the ability to hold aromas and flavours.

Are fats, hard in consistency?

The hardness of fat is determined by its fatty acids. Fatty acids containing [illegible]lve carbon atoms or fewer are liquid at room temperature. Saturated fatty acids containing fourteen carbon atoms are solid at room temperature.

Animal fats are saturated containing 30 to 60 percent saturated fatty acids containing stearic and palmitic acid. In general hervivore have harder fats than carnivore. Land animals have harder fats than aquatic animals.

The proportion of saturated fatty acids is high in milk fat, but this fat is soft.

Can fats be emulsified?

Fats are capable of forming emulsions with liquids thus increasing the surface area and reducing the surface tension. Quality of emulsification is utilized in homogenization of milk and in preparing mayonnaise.

What do you understand by Saponification?

The combination of a fatty acid by a cation to form a soap is known by saponification. In the alkaline medium of intestine, calcium is to form insoluble compound being excreted in feces.

How heating affects fat?

Excessive heating of fats leads to the breakdown of glycerol, producing a pungent compound acrolein which is irritating to stomach. Fatty acids are oxidized by prolonged heating at room temperature.

How fats become rancid?

At room temperature air can induce oxidation of fats making it rancid. In this odor and flavour is changed. Unsaturated fats become rancid easily. Some fats are naturally protected by presence of antioxidants like vitamin E.

What are the functions of fat?

All body cells contain some fat. Body contains 15 to 20% of fat. With age proportion of fat increases.

Cell membranes contain lipids that facilitate transfer of nutrients.

How many calories one gram of fat provides?

Primary aim of fat is to give calories. Each gram of fat when oxidized gives 9 calories more than twice of protein or carbohydrates. High density and low solubility of fats make them fit to be stored.

A woman of 55 Kg of which 20 percent to fat has a store of 85,000 K cal. She can survive for 30-40 days.

What is the satiety role of fat?

Fats reduce gastric motility and remain in stomach longer so sensation of hunger is delayed. Fats have higher satiety level. Flavour of many fruits is due to volatile oils.

How fats helps in insulation and padding of body organs?

The subcutaneous layer of fat is an effective insulator and reduces loss of body heat. Vital organs and kidney are protected by a pad of fat.

Are fats effective carrier of fat soluble vitamins?

Fat is a carrier of fat soluble vitamin ADEK. Some fat is necessary for absorption of vitamin A precursor carotene.

What are phospholipids?

All cells contain phospholipids. But brain, nervous tissue and liver are rich in them. Phospholipids are powerful emulsifying agent and have an affinity for water. These are essential to the digestion and absorption of fats. They facilitate the uptake of fatty acids by the cells.

What is cholesterol?

It is a component of cell membrane and furnishes the nucleus for synthesis of provitamin D, adrenocortical hormones, steroid sex hormones and bile salts.

The concentration of cholesterol is high in liver, adrenals, white/gray matter of brain and peripheral nerves.

Are fats precursors of protaglandins?

In 1962 substances stimulating the contraction of smooth muscles in the walls of blood vessels were identified as prostaglandins. Prostaglandins perform following functions –

- Promoting conception and inducing labour.
- Spontaneous abortions
- Regulating transmission of nerve impulses.
- Inhibiting lipolysis and gastric secretion.
- Maintains blood pressure.

Are fats source of essential fatty acids?

Yes, among the fatty acid is a polyunsaturated fatty acid, linoleic acid which is effective in curing dermatitis. Linoleic acid is present in vegetable oils such as corn oil, sunflower oil containing 50% linoleic acid.

What are the fatty acid content of certain oils?

Fatty acid contents in percentage

	% Fat	Saturated Fat	Oleic Acid	Linoleic Acid
Safflower	100	10	13	74
Sunflower	100	9	12	74
Corn oil	100	10	20	65
Soya bean	100	14	23	50
Peanut	100	17	45	32
Olive	100	14	73	8
Palm oil	100	81	11	2
Butter	81	61	20	2
Animal fats	100	30	37	20
Peanut butter	51	17	46	32
Egg yolk	33	10	12	4
Coconut	100	86	6	2
Seasame	100	14	30	41

How is fat digested?

Almost all fats presented to digestive tract are triglycerides. Fats are hydrolysed primarily in small intestine although gastric lipase brings about some hydrolysis of finely divided fats. Long chain fatty acids are less likely to be attacked by lipase.

Most of digestion of fat takes place in intestine. Here bilesalts arrange themselves on the surface of unemulsified triglycerides to break them into very small particles. The pancreatic lipase attacks each triglyceride molecule and release the fatty acid.

What is the speed of digestion of fats?

High fats remain longer in stomach than diet in low fat. Fats which are liquid at body temperature are hydrolysed more rapidly than those solid at body temperature. Infants and old may experience some discomfort following meals high in fat. If frying temperature is too low food absorbs excessive amounts of fat which lengthens the time for digestion.

How fats are absorbed?

In small intestine the free fatty acids, monoglycerides, some diglycerides and triglycerides are absorbed.

Fatty acids are absorbed into portal circulation. They are attached to albumin for their transportation and may be used in liver or released to other tissues in body.

Normally about 95% of dietary fats and 10 to 50% of dietary cholesterol are absorbed.

What are the factors which reduce absorption of fat?

A number of factors reduce the amount of fat that is digested and absorbed as

- Increased intestinal motility not giving sufficient time for action of enzymes.
- Diseases of biliary tract so that secretion of bile is deficient.
- Diseases of pancreas so that lipase is not secreted.

When fat absorption is decreased large amount of fats are excreted.

What are the blood levels of lipids?

In normal person cholesterol concentration ranges from 150 to 225 mg per 100 ml. Preferred level is below 200 mg.

The normal triglycerides level after 12 hour fast is 140 mg/100 ml.

However cholesterol and triglycerides don't exist in the free state in circulation. Since fats are insoluble in water proteins provide mechanism for their transport. These protein lipid complexes are known as lipoproteins.

What are low density lipids?

Two broad classes have been described. Very low density lipoproteins (VL DL) contain a high proportion of triglycerides and a small amount of protein. When this is elevated there is possibility of carbohydrate induced hyperlipidemia.

Low density lipoproteins (LDL) are the chief carriers of cholesterol and are relatively low in glycerides. The concentration of this increases with age and with diets rich in fatty acids.

What about high density lipoproteins?

These consist of about 50% protein and 20% cholesterol. This group is protective to heart and reduces risk of coronary heart disease.

What are free fatty acids?

These are known as nonsterified fatty acids. These are the principal source of fatty acids made available to the cells for energy. They enter the circulation as the result of hydrolysis of triglycerides chiefly by adipose tissue. The concentration of FFA in the blood at any given time is low. But level is higher in the circulation during fasting.

How adipose tissue is related with fat metabolism?

The adipose cell is a specialised cells that provides for the synthesis, storage and release of fats. Fat synthesis and breakdown takes place continuously.

When a calorie deficiency exists the adipose tissue will be catabolised more rapidly than it is being synthesize.

How liver helps in fat metabolism?

Liver is the main organ in regulation of fat metabolism. The liver hydrolyses the triglycerides brought to it, reforms new triglycerides and again releases to them to circulation. It also synthesizes triglycerides from free fatty acids and glucose.

Phospholipids and lipoproteins are synthesized and released to the circulation or removed from circulation maintaining control over blood levels.

Liver is the chief regulater of total body content of cholesterol and of circulating blood cholesterol.

What are lipotropic substances?

Certain lipotropic substances must be present to prevent the accumulation of fat in liver. They include choline, vitamin B12 and inositol.

What about synthesis of fats?

Triglycerides are synthesized by epithelial cells of intestinal mucosa, by the adipose tissue and by liver. In order to synthesize triglycerides a source of glycerophosphate is essential which is furnished by normal oxidation of glucose.

What about ketogenesis?

Within liver two molecules of acetyl coenzyme A can condense to form acetoacetyl coenzyme which in turn yields acetoacetic acid and acetone. These compounds are known as ketone bodies and process is known as ketogenesis. Muscles and other cells can utilize to yield energy.

But during weight reduction ketones are produced more in uncontrolled diabetes mellitus. Ketosis occurs because of lack of insulin for the metabolism of carbohydrate.

Describe cholesterol metabolism?

Liver and intestines are the chief sites of cholesterol synthesis although all cells are capable to produce some cholesterol. Within body 800-1500 mg of cholesterol is produced independent of dietary supplement.

Cholesterol is transported in the blood in various classes of lipoproteins. Body is unable to breakdown cholesterol nucleus. Only liver can convert it by enzyme action to bile acid. Excretion occurs through intestine.

Showing cholesterol content of foods mg/100 gm.

Food	Cholesterol	Food	Cholesterol
Butter	280	Egg white	0
Cheese	145	Egg yolk	1330
Cream	140	Chicken	40
Milk	11	Liver	250
Egg hen	498	Fish	50

What is the dietary requirement of fat?

A diet providing 2% of its calories from linoleic acid meets the requirement 25% to 35% of total calories may be derived from fats. In gall bladder diseases total 10% calories may be derived from fats.

What is the relationship of higher consumption of fat and heart disease?

High cholesterol level people are at high risk of heart attack. It is a major constituent of atheromatous plaque. These plaques narrow the diameter of arteries but dietary control of cholesterol does not give good results every time. Since a certain amount of cholesterol is vital for the synthesis of sex hormones, a precursor of vitamin D and A component of all cell membrane.

What are the rich dietary sources of fat?

Showing important sources of fat

Food	% Fat	Food	% Fat
Ghee	100	Soyabean	19.5
Butter	81	Cow's milk	3.5
Almond	58.9	Egg	13.3
Cashew nut	46	Mutton	13.3
Ground nut	40	Fish	3.2

White portion of an egg is full of proteins and yellow portion full of cholesterol. If you are keen to avoid fats consume low fats, skimmed milk, green vegetables, fruits and pulses.

What are oils?

For centuries vital oils have been known for their skin softening and good source of vitamin ADE and K. Vitamin E and certain fatty acids are required to maintain skin's elasticity. This delays aging by slowing down wrinkles.

Olive oil can easily be incorporated in daily diet.

Cod liver oil is a rich source of vitamin A & D. It is very useful to treat rickets.

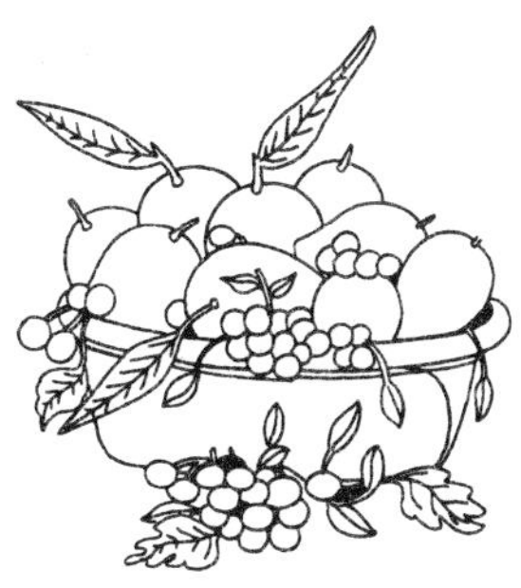

Carbohydrates

Carbohydrates are the most abundant compounds in universe. Cellulose which makes up the structured parts of plants accounts for about half the carbon in vegetation. Plants are valued for their large stores of starches/sugars.

What is the composition of carbohydrates?

These are simple sugars or polymers of sugars such as starch that can be hydrolysed to simple sugars by action of digestive enzymes or on heating with dilute acid.

How carbohydrates can be classified?

Carbohydrates can be classified as

(i) Monosaccharide

(ii) Disaccharide

(iii) Polysaccharide

Monosaccharides are compounds that cannot be hydrolised to simpler compounds.

What is glucose?

It is a monosaccharide and is known as dextrose, grape sugar or corn sugar. It is found is grapes, berries and oranges. Some vegetables such as sweet corn and carrots also contain it. It is the end product of di and polysaccharide. It is utilized by cell for energy.

What is fructose?

Levulose or fruit sugar is a highly soluble sugar which does not crystallize. It is much sweeter than sugar and is found in honey, ripe fruits and some vegetables.

Describe disaccharides?

In it two hexoses are combined with the loss of one molecule of water. The emperical formula is $C_{12} H_{22} O_{11}$. They are water soluble, diffusible and crystallizable. They can be split into simple sugars by acid hydrolysis.

(i) Sucrose is the table sugar and is found in sugarcane or beet sugar. Many fruits and some vegetables contain small amount of sucrose.

(ii) Lactose or milk sugar is produced by mammals and is only carbohydrate from animal source. Its content in milk varies from 2 to 8%.

(iii) Maltose does not occur in sufficient quantity in foods. It is an intermediary product in the hydrolysis of starch. It is used in some infant formulas.

What are polysaccharides?

These are complex compounds with relatively high molecular weight. These are not sweet and are insoluble in water. Starch, dextrins, glycogen are of clinical interest.

(i) Dextrins are intermediate products in the hydrolysis of starch and consists of shorter chains. Some dextrins is produced when toast is made of bread.

(ii) Glycogen is 'animal starch' and contains many more branched chains of glucose. It is rapidly synthesized from glucose in the liver and muscle.

(iii) Starch – It is the storage form of carbohydrate and is an important source of energy. It has two types of glucose chains

a. Amylase

b. Armylopectine

Armylopectin has colloidal properties so that thickening of a starch water mixture occurs when it is heated.

What are insoluble polysaccharides?

These include cellulose, hemicellulose, pectin, gums and mucilage.

What are carbohydrate derivatives?

Sugars react chemically to form sugar alcohol, aminosugars, glycosides

- Glycerol is the 3-carbon alcohol that is a component of glycerides.
- Sorbitol is sweet, it is sugar alcohol, water soluble and found in cherries, plums and berries.
- Inositol is an alcohol related to hexoses. It occurs in bran of cereal grains. When it combines with phosphate it forms phytic acid a compound that interferes with the absorption of minerals such as calcium, iron and zinc.

What is the distribution of carbohydrate in body?

The amount of carbohydrate in the adult body is about 300-350 gram. Of this 100 gram is stored as glycogen in liver. Another 200-250 gm is present as glycogen in cardiac, smooth and skeletal muscles.

Rest of 15 gram of glucose lies in blood and extracellular fluid.

In what different forms carbohydrate lies in body?

- Hyaluronic acid, a viscous substance forms matrix of connective tissue.
- Heparin in substance which prevents clotting of blood.

- Chondroitin sulfates found in skin, tendons, cartilage, bone and heart valves.
- DNA and RNA which transfer the genetic characteristic of cell.
- Glycosides as components of steroid and adrenal hormones.

How are carbohydrates used as source of energy?

Each gram of carbohydrate gives 4.1 calories. These are the cheapest source of calories. Glucose is the primary source of energy for lungs and nervous system.

Total glycogen reserves in body would meet about half of one days energy. Glycogen in muscles can be used to supply energy needs of muscle cells but is not available for regulation of blood sugar level.

What is the protein sparing action of carbohydrates?

The body will first use carbohydrates as a source of energy when it is adequately supplied, hence proteins remains spared for body building. But if there is any deficiency of carbohydrates then protein and fats will be utilised for calories.

Are carbohydrates needed in regulation of fat metabolism?

Some carbohydrates are needed in diet so that oxidation of fats can proceed normally. In absence of carbohydrates fats will be metabolised faster and accumulation of incompletely oxidized products will lead to dehydration, loss of sodium and ketosis. At least 50 grams of carbohydrates are needed to avoid ketoacidosis.

What is the role of carbohydrates in G.I.T. functions?

Lactose promotes the growth of desirable bacteria, some of which are useful in synthesis of B-complex vitamins. Lactose enhances the absorption of calcium.

Dietary fibres don't yield energy but helps in peristaltic movements and does not permit constipation to develop.

How carbohydrates are digested?

The main purpose of digestion is to hydrolyse di and polysaccharides of the diet to simple sugars. Certain enzymes help in digestion.

Starch	+	amylase	→	Glucose
Sucrose	+	sucrase	→	Glucose + fructose
Maltose	+	maltase	→	Glucose + glucose
Lactose	+	Lactose	→	Glusoce + galactose

Some hydrolysis of starch to maltose occurs in mouth by salivary amylase. Main site of digestion of carbohydrate is small intestine.

Salivary amylase does not act upon raw starch but pancreatic amylase hydrolyses both row and cooked starch to dextrins maltose. Cooked starch is more rapidly hydrolysed.

How carbohydrates are absorbed?

Simple sugars enter the epithelial cell, transported across the cell, enter interstitial fluid and pass through the blood capillaries for transport to portal circulation and liver to be dispensed according to the need to the systemic circulation.

Glucose and galactose can be absorbed by passive diffusion.

What is the role of Liver in carbohydrate metabolism?

Monosaccharides are carried by the portal vein to the liver. The liver converts galactose and fructose to glucose. It synthesizes glycogen from glucose, stores it and reconverts to glucose if the glycogen stores are depleted. It can transform excess glucose into fatty acids.

How blood glucose level is maintained?

By means of blood circulation glucose is made continuously available to each and every cell of body as a source of energy. Glucose taken from circulation by cells is constantly replaced by the liver so that blood glucose level is maintained.

In the fasting state blood glucose concentration is normally 60 to 85 mg percent. Shortly after meal it rises to 140 to 150 mg but after 2 hours comes to normal. If it crosses 180 mg it may pass in urine. It is known as renal threshold and depends from man to man.

What do you understand by glycolysis?

Chemical reaction takes place in the cytoplasmic matrix of cell. This reaction degrade glucose to pyruvic acid in preparation of entrance into mitrochondria. The entrance of glucose into the cell is facilitated by insulin.

What is the role of lactic acid?

Pyruvic acid can proceed anaerobically to form lactic acid which is utilized for muscle contraction under condition when energy needs exceeds the supply of O_2.

FIBRES

What is fibre and why it is important?

Fibre is the skeleton of plant. The walls of every cell are composed of fibre. Fibre is more abundant outsides the seeds, fruits, legumes and other foods. Milling and peeling removes all fibre. Fibre is also removed when the content of cell is extracted and cell wall removed just like getting sugar out of sugar cane.

What are the components of fibre?

Fibre is not a single substance but is basically a mixture of 3 main groups.

(i) Cellulose

(ii) Lignin

(iii) Pectin

Previously fibre was thought to be only cellulose which is really the least important part. Crude fibre is not broken down even if boiled in weak acid or weak alkali.

What is the simplest definition of fibre?

It is the part of plant food which passes through the small intestine almost entirely undigested and reaches the large intestine relatively intact, while other starches, sugars and protein eaten are digested and absorbed through small intestine.

What happens to fiber in body?

Fiber does not provide much of calories. Fibre in stomach delays the absorption of energy largely in form of glucose. In the small and large intestine fibre interacts with cholesterol and bile salts. In large intestine fibre provides food for bacteria which are beneficial to body. The smooth muscular movements of large bowel and the passage of soft fairy large feces depends on whether there bacteria get sufficient to eat in the form of fibre.

Lack of fibre, and of cereal fibre in particular is the most important single cause of constipation. If fibre intake are adequate, laxative will be rarely required.

What effect does dietary fibre have on stools?

When diet is very rich in fibre stool passed are usually large in volume, pale in colour, soft in consistency and stool often floats in water. Softness of fibre is due to presence of emulsified gas produced by action of bacteria on fibre. Any amount of water, fruit, and vegetables don't help much in treating constipation.

What are the rich source of dietary fibres?

Total dietary fibre in 100 gm of food

Food	% of fibre
Bran	48.0
Whole wheat flour	11.7
Peas	7.7
Carrots	3.7
Cabbage	2.9
Banana	1.8
Plum	1.5
Apple	1.4
Tomatoes	1.4

How fibre helps in diverticulosis?

Diverticular disease is the development of small pouches blown through the wall of colon. Constipation is the primary cause. When fecal material is firm in consistency it puts more pressure to proper fecal material. In bargain some portion bulges out. So the small, hard dried stools associated with constipation lead to diverticula formation then the aim must be to encourage large, soft, moist stools which can be achieved by eating more fibre.

How high fibre diet can avoid appendicitis?

Appendicitis is the inflammation of appendix. Infection comes after blockage of cavity of appendix. Mostly a small hard lump of fecal matter about the size of pea is found causing blockage. In certain studies there has been found inverse relationship between fibre intake and appendicitis.

Are fibres useful in piles?

Main cause of piles is hard stool. When stool is hard the straining necessary for its evacuation forces piles to bleed. High fibre diet keeps the stool soft.

What are the important source of carbohydrates?

Carbohydrate contents of food

Food	Gram/100 gram
Bread	50-55
Wheat flour	71-80
Legumes dry	60-65
Nuts	15-20
Potatoes	17
Rice dry	70
Biscuits	51-60
Fruit dried	59-69
Ice cream	18-21
Milk	5
Sugar	96-100
Vegetable	4-18

What will happen when you consume low carbohydrates?

Very low carbohydrate diets can cause ketosis with excessive fatigue, dehydration, water loss and electrolyte. There may be retention of uric acid giving rise to gout. Low carbohydrate diets are low in fibre too.

What will happen if carbohydrates are high in diet?

A high proportion of calories from carbohydrate is desirable if diet is furnished by complex carbohydrate. Sugar is useful as concentrated source of energy but should not provide more than 10% of calories. Too much consumption of sugar may crowd out essential food. If you consume lot of soft drinks you may not take milk or so.

Can rich carbohydrate diet produce dental caries?

Yes, sugar provides the energy for bacterial growth, which leads to gradual build up of plaque, a sticky carbohydrate bacterial matrix that adheres to the teeth. The acid formed by bacteria from sugar substrate gradually erode the tooth enamel and bring out decay. Two conditions accelerate the process, sticky carbohydrate and frequent exposure of tooth to sugars.

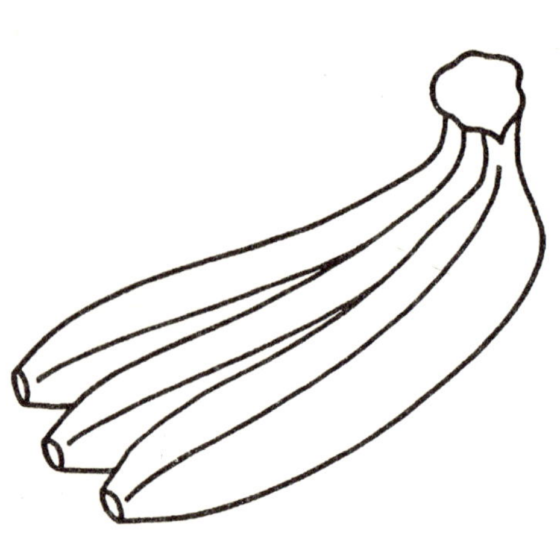

What are sugar substitutes?

Those who are obese and wants to enjoy sweet foods low calories sweetening agents are available such as fructose, aspartame, a dipeptide and saccharine.

What is aspartame?

It is 160 times more sweater than sucrose. It may be used as a table top sweetener in preparing tea, puddings, halwa etc. Because it contains one of two aminoacids it must be avoided by individuals suffering from phenylketonuria. Since it is degraded at high temperature it is not suitable for cooked preparation.

What is marginine?

It is of bitter taste and is found in rind of grapes. It can be converted into a substance which is 1500 more sweeter than sugar and three times that of saccharin. It is stable at high temperature.

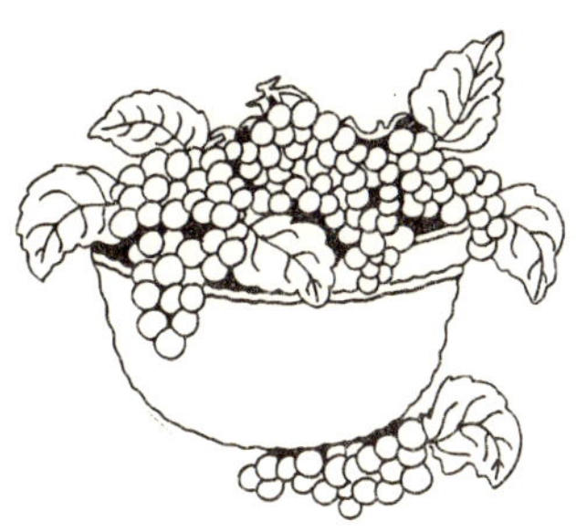

Calories

What are the different forms of energy?

Energy is the capacity to do work. The potential energy is transformed to other forms to do work of body. Mechanical energy is needed for muscle contraction, osmotic energy to transport fluids and nutrients, electrical energy for transmission of nerve impulses. Thermal energy is required for heat regulation and chemical energy for synthesis of new compounds.

What is the unit of calories?

Kilo calorie is the amount of heat required to raise the temperature of 1 Kg water 1^0C from 15^0 to 16^0 centigrade. It is 1000 times higher than small calorie used in physics.

What is Joules?

Joule is the unit of energy used in metric system. It is the amount of energy expanded when 1 Kg is moved a distance of 1 meter by a force of 1 Newton. It is equal to 107 ergs. It is an energy expressed in mechanical equivalent, not heat equivalent.

Following factors apply for the interconversion of calories and joules

1 calorie	=	4.184 J
1 Kcal	=	4184 MJ
1 MJ	=	240 Kcal

What is the law of conversation of energy?

Whenever one form of energy is produced another form is reduced by the same amount. This is law of conservation of energy. It states that energy neither can be destroyed nor created. When food supplys more energy than needed by body rest is stored as fat resulting in weight gain. This stored energy can be used when needed.

How food calories are estimated?

Fuel values of food are easily determined by means of an instrument known as Bomb calorimeter. A weighed amount of dried food is placed in a heavy steel container bomb. The bomb is placed in well insulated vessel and is surrounded by a well known volume of water. The sample is ignited and heat is dissipated into water. By noting the change in temperature of water one can calculate the energy value of food.

BASAL METABOLIC RATE

What is basal metabolic rate?

The amount of energy required to carry on the involuntary work of body is known as basal metabolic rate. Involuntary work includes the functional activity of different vital organs brain, heart, lungs, glands and peristaltic movement of intestines. Some energy is also required for maintenance of muscle tone and body temperature. Brain and nervous system require 1/5 th of energy and other organs 3/5 th of energy.

Under what conditions BMR is estimated?

- It is performed in the morning 12-16 hours after last meal.
- One hour of rest in lying down position
- Relaxed and free emotional environment.
- Normal body temperature.
- Room temperature should be comfortable about 21^0 to 24^0C.

What is indirect calorimetery?

It measures the amount of oxygen consumed in a given time period. 1 liter of oxygen is equal to 4.825 Kcal. The energy expenditure at varying levels of activity can be measured by a respirometer under controlled condition either walking on tread mill or on a stationary cycle.

How much is BMR?

This is 40 calories per hour per square meter of body surface in males and 37 in females.

Taking the area of an adult as 1.75 square meters basic calorie requirement comes to

40 X 1.75 X 24 = 1700

It accounts to 60% of total energy requirement.

Does BMR depends on body surface area?

Yes, 80 percent of energy from glucose and fat is lost as heat and 15% from skin. Remaining heat loss occurs from lungs and through excreta.

Metabolic rate is directly related with body size.

Does woman requires less of calories?

Woman have a metabolic rate about 6 to 10% lower than that of man. The influence of sex hormone may account for some of difference.

How age affects BMR?

BMR is highest in life for first 2 years of life than it declines and accelerates slightly in adolescence. Then it decreases 2% for every decade. Rapid growth rate explains the high BMR. In older age group lessened muscle tone and reduction in muscle mass account for lower rate.

Does BMR fall during sleep?

During sleep hours the BMR is about 10% lower than day hours.

How body temperature affects BMR?

An elevation of body temperature increases BMR. A rise of 1^0F in body temperature leads to an average increase of 7% in BMR. Rise of temperature by 1^0C increases BMR by 13%. Hence person in fever develops high BMR and requires more calories.

How hormone secretions affect BMR?

Thyroid and adrenals have more influence on BMR. In hypothyroidism BMR may even go down by 30% Hyperthyroidism may elevate basal needs by 50 to 70%.

During emotional stress of anger or fear epinephrine is produced which raises BMR for 2-3 hours.

Does pregnancy affects BMR?

During the last trimester of pregnancy there is an increase in BMR by 20%. This may be due to high activity of fetus and placenta.

Is resting metabolism and BMR the same?

No, resting metabolism should be differentiated from BMR. It applies to energy expenditure under normal life condition while at rest. It takes into the account of minimum metabolism at night and during day when there is no exercise.

What is calorie expenditure during sedentary type of work?

Sedentary work includes reading, writing, watching T.V. listening to radio, playing cards. Expenditure of calories is in between 80 to 100/hour.

What will be the calorie expenditure during light work?

Light work includes cooking food, dusting, personal care, walking slow. Expenditure of calories is 110 to 160 calories/hour.

What includes moderate activity?

Mopping, scrubbing, sweeping, laundry, carpenter work, fast walking all come under moderate activity and it requires 170 to 240 calories per hour.

What is strenuous activity?

Swimming, playing tennis, dancing, running requires 350 and more calories per hour.

Does mental work requires extra calories?

Nervous system is continuously active and its energy requirement is 20% of BMR. Even very hard mental exercise does not require extra calories.

What are the ICMR recommendation of calories?

Nutrition advisory committee (1958) of ICMR has suggested the following values for each type of work.

Light work	1.7 calories/kg/hour
Moderate work	2.5 calories/kg/hour
Heavy work	5 calories/kg/hour

Do woman require more calories during pregnancy?

Extra energy is needed during stages of rapid growth of building tissues. These include pregnancy, and adolescence. Total energy need for pregnancy is estimated to be 40,000 kilo calories. To secrete 700 ml milk for an infant mother's extra need of energy is 600-700 per day.

What are the daily recommended allowances for calories?

Table showing daily allowances for calories.

Individual	Calories/day
• Man (55 kg)	
Sedentary work	2400
Moderate work	2800
Heavy work	3900
• Woman (45 kg)	
Sedentary work	1900
Moderate work	2200
Heavy work	3000
Pregnancy (second half)	+ 300
Lactation	+ 700
•Infants/Children	
0-6 months	120/ kg
7-12 months	100/kg
1-3 years	1200
4-6 years	1600
7-9 years	1800
10-12 years	2100
• Girls	
13-15 years	2000
16-18 years	2200
• Boys	
13-15 years	2500
16-18 years	3000

In a group of different age groups how will you calculate the energy requirement?

With the scale of coefficient one can calculate the energy requirement of a group.

Person	Coefficient
• Adult male	
Sedentary work	1.0
Moderate work	1.2
Heavy work	1.6
• Adult female	
Sedentary work	0.8
Moderate work	0.9
Heavy work	1.2
19-21 years	1.0
9-12	0.8
7-9	0.7
5-7	0.6
3-5	0.5
1-3	0.4

For example a family of mother

father and two children 10 and 4 years of age . The minimum daily requirement of calories will be. 7200.

0.8 + 1 + 0.7 + 0.5 = 3 i.e 2400 X 3 = 7200

On what factors energy requirement depends?

- 75% Human energy requirement is directly proportional

to body size and 25% on body weight.

- Below 14^{0}C increase of 5% calories are needed in carrying more clothings or counter shivering.
- Above 30^{0}C = 80^{0}F have an increased calorie need of 0.5% for each degree in environmental temperature.
- Adjustment of calories for activity and during pregnancy has to be made.

What is calorie imbalance?

As long as calorie intake is equal to calorie expenditure body weight remains normal. Persons whose intake constantly exceeds their expenditure soon becomes concious of storage of calories in the form of body weight due to deposition of fats. Persons whose intake is inadequate, start loosing weight. For every 3500 Kcal deficit in diet 0.5 kg body fat will be oxidized or lost or vice versa. It does not matter whether imbalance is one of 700 Kcal for each five days or 10 Kcal for 350 days. The end result is the same.

LIQUID CALORIES

What are liquid calories?

Most of the people think that solid foods are fattening and liquid food contains low calories but it is not always so.

Are fruit juices very low in calories?

Caloric value of different fruit juices.

Fruit	Average measure	Quantity ml	Calories
Apple	1 glass	240	120
Pine apple	1 glass	240	140
Grape	1 glass	240	170
Orange	1 glass	240	110
Lemon	1 glass	240	73+

What about soft drinks?

Most soft drink exceed in food calories. A 300 ml of soft drink will contain about 120-140 calories. Each bottle contain 6 tea spoonful of sugars. Most of the soft drinks contains sodium which increases the requirement of water. Now a days low calorie drinks are also available in market.

Does soda contains lot of calories?

No, soda hardly contains any calories. These are just carbonated water containing sweeteners and preservatives.

What about various drinks containing milk?

Calorie content will depend on the fat contents of milk, sugar, and calories of chocolates or Horlicks.

Preparation	Average measure	Quantity	Calories
Whole milk	1 glass	240 ml	192
Cocoa + milk	1 glass	240 ml	230
Chocolate milk	1 glass	240 ml	270
Horlicks 2TSF + TSF sugar	1 glass	240 ml	325
Coffee	1 tea cup		76
Tea	1 tea cup		60

The perfect low calorie drink who are dieting is butter milk, coconut water. One bowl of 240 ml of thick tomato soup contains 90 calories plain. Water does not contain any calories.

What about alcohol?

Each gram of alcohol gives you 7 empty calories and contains zero nutrient.

On the other hand liquor depletes the body of nutrients as it hampers the absorption of zinc, vitamin C and vitamin B complex. It increases production of HCL and gastric juices and works as a appetiser. Snacks generally consumed with drinks adds to your calorie consumption.

Does alcohol requires more of water to be consumed?

Yes, body requires eight ounces of water to metabolize one ounce of alcohol. Water for this is derived from the cells and therefore tongue becomes dry. Alcohol dehydrates the skin making a more prone to wrinkles when taken on an empty stomach. Food and fats consumed side by side hampers alcohol absorption.

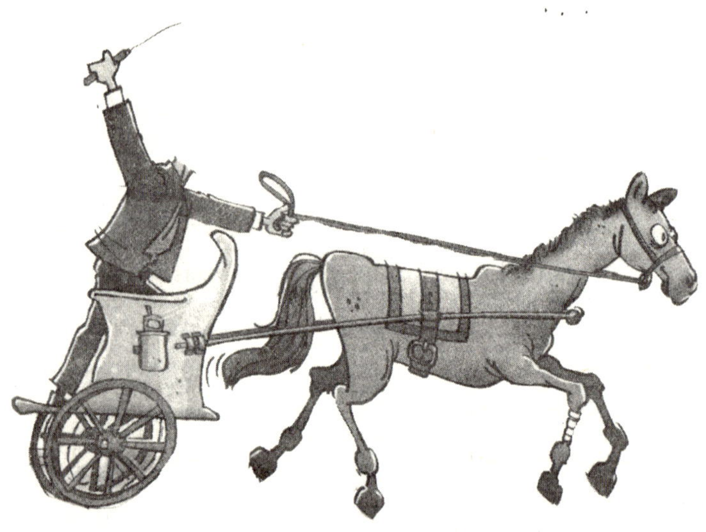

What are the average calories of different alcoholic beverages?

Drink	Average measure	Quantity ml	Calories
Beer	1 glass	240	100
Brandy	1 ounce	30	23
Gin	1.5 ounce	43	105
Whisky	1.5 ounce	43	120
Toddy	1 glass	240	144
Wine	1 wine glass	120	170
Sherry	1 wine glass	120	145

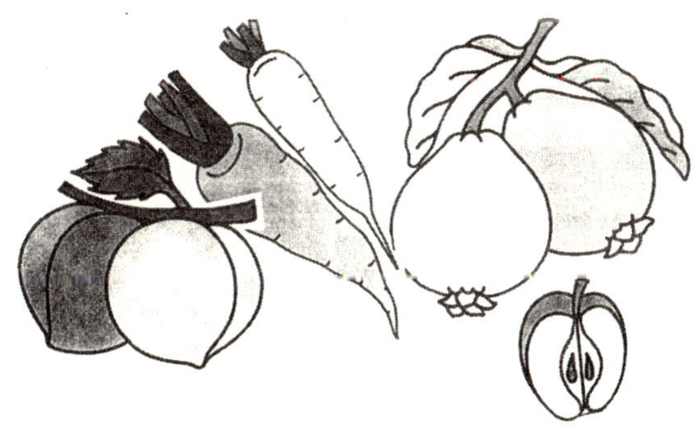

Vitamins

What are vitamins?

Vitamins are defined as organic substances needed in very small amount performing a specific metabolic function and must be provided in diet from outside. Body cannot synthesize them.

How the term 'vitamin' was coined?

It was coined by Casimir Funk in 1912. He found out that bran can cure beriberi. Vita = necessary for life and amine = nitrogen containing hence the term vitamin which protects pellagra, scurvy and rickets. Later on was found that all were containing 'amine' so the final 'e' was dropped giving the familiar term vitamin.

What are provitamins?

Precursors are substances that are chemically related to biologically active form of vitamin but have no vitamin activity until the body converts them into active form. Carotenes are converted into vitamin A in the intestine wall. Tryptophan is converted to niacin in liver.

Are there antivitamins also?

Vitamin antagonists or pseudovitamins are usually chemically related to biologically active vitamin. There are used to produce vitamin deficiencies.

How vitamins are measured?

Previously potency of vitamins could be measured only by their ability to promote growth or to cure a deficiency when test doses are fed to experimental animals. Such measurements are known as bioassay and has been expressed in units. Vitamin A.D.E and K are expressed in units.

Other vitamins are measured by their ability to promote the growth of microorganisms known as microbiologic assay in units of weight in mgm or microgram. The weight of ascorbic acid is 20,000 times that of vitamins B12.

How vitamins have been classified?

These have been divided into two.

- Water soluble vitamins are
- Vitamin C
- Vitamin B complex

Thiamine (B1) Pyridoxin (B6)

Niacin Biotin

Riboflavin Cyanocobalamine (B12)

Folate

What are the general properties of fat soluble and water soluble vitamins?

Fat Soluble Vitamins	Water Soluble
Soluble in fat and fat solvent	Soluble in water
Excessive intake will be deposited in body	Minimal storage
Small amount excreted in bile	Excreted in urine
Not to be in diet every day	Requires every day
Have provitamins	Don't have provitamins
Absorbed in lymphatic system	Absorbed in blood
Needed only by complexed organism	Needed by mostly simple and complex organisms

Is there any difference in natural and synthetic vitamins?

Natural vitamins are biochemically identical to those produced, synthetically and are absorbed exactly the same way. So there is no difference between the two. Advertisements for natural vitamins are misleading.

Can over consumption of vitamins be toxic?

Excessive consumption of water soluble vitamins are excreted unchanged in urine so problem of toxicity don't arise. One can take ten folds of requirement of vitamins. While fat soluble vitamins get deposited in body and cause toxic effects.

VITAMIN – A

When vitamin A was invented?

In 1912 Osborne and Mendel reported that animals grow normally on milk diet but in absence of milk growth failure is followed by eye disease. By 1928 carotene one of yellow pigments of plants had been identified as precursor of vitamin A.

What are the units of vitamin A?

Until 1967 vitamin A activity were expressed in International units I.U. In 1967 retinol equivalent 'R.E' was introduced. One RE is equal to 1 mg of retinol, 6 mg of beta carotene and 12 mg of other carotenoid precursor. When vitamin A is expressed in I.U., one retinol equals 3.33 I.U. retional and 10 I.U. beta carotene.

What are the characteristics of vitamin A?

Vitamin A is a pale yellow substance. It is soluble in fat or fat solvent. With the exception of spinach the preformed biologically active form of vitamin A is found only in animal foods.

What is Beta-carotene?

Beta carotene, a vitamin A precursor with a pronounced yellow colour in its purified form was produced in 1954. It is one of few pigments permitted to colour the food.

How vitamin A is absorbed?

Vitamin A changes many forms before it is absorbed. Pancreatic juice splits it to form free retinol. Bile is needed for uptake of retinol by mucosal cells. It combines with fatty acid usually palmitic and incorporated in small transport particles of fat chylomicrons. Almost all retinol and 33% carotene is absorbed. These are than released into lymphatic circulation which eventually goes to liver through blood circulation.

Vitamin E enhances absorption and increases the amount stored in liver. While liver injury and bile duct obstruction decreases it.

What is the relation of vision and vitamin A?

Vitamin A is related to the maintenance of normal vision in dim light. Retina contains Rods and Cones. Rods are responsible for vision in dim light and cones are responsible for vision in bright and colour vision. In both these pigments vitamin A is present.

How vitamin A helps epithelial tissues?

Vitamins A is required for healthy epithelium. Vitamin A gives protection against infection, but large intake of vitamin A will not confer additional protective benefits.

What are the other functions of vitamin A?

Vitamin A is essential for normal skeletal and tooth development. With a deficiency of vitamin A bones don't grow in length and normal remodelling process does not take place. Exact process is not known.

Vitamin A is necessary for spermatogenesis in male and normal estrus cycle in female. If sufficient vitamin A is not available fetal malformation may result. Vitamin 'A' is needed for iron metabolism.

What is the daily allowance of vitamin A?

The vitamin A allowance for boys is 1,000 RD or 5,000 I.U. and for females over 10 years it is 800 RE or 4000 I.U. The allowances for infants over 6 months to 10 years are 400-700 RE, pregnancy 1000 RE and for lactation 1200 RE.

What are the food sources of vitamin A?

Food	Vitamin A I.U.	Retinol equivalent
Spinach ½ cup	10,600	1060
Carrots sliced ½ cup	9065	906
Peas ½ cup	575	58
Bean ½ cup		
Papaya ½ cup	1595	160
Peaches Raw ½ cup	1115	112
Orange 1 medium	290	29
Banana 1 medium	95	10
Pine apple ½ cup	90	9
Milk 1 cup	390	118
Cheese 1 ounce	378	114
Butter 1 table spoon	230	70
Egg whole	590	179
Beef 3 ounces fever	45450	13773
Chicken	27000	8182
Pork	12000	3636

Egg yolk with 3300 I.U. or 1000 RE/100 gm is a good source of vitamin A in the form of retinol. A deep yellow colour may reflect unconverted carotene.

In milk vitamin A is present in fat portion and is absent in non fat milk. Dried nonfat milk solids are fortified with vitamin A. Any yellow colour in milk like cows milk contains carotene. Amount of vitamin A in cheese is same as that in milk.

Fruits and vegetables contains no preformed vitamin A, only precursors. Yellow pigment in corn, cryptoxanthin does have vitamin A potential of about 3.5 I.U/gram.

Signs of vitamin A deficiency.

Once liver stores of vitamin A are depleted signs of vitamin A deficiency symptoms may develop due to (I) low dietary intakes (ii) interference with conversion of carotene (iii) rapid loss of vitamin A.

Can vitamin A deficiency lead to night blindness?

It is one of 'the earliest symptom. Low level results in drop in vitamin A level available in retina of eye needed for formation of visual pigment odopsin.

What other changes in eye develops due to vitamin A deficiency?

The lacrimal gland fails to secrete tears. Dry eye results as a consequence. There develops sloughing of epithelial cells of cornea. Infection sets in. Bitol's spot develop. Total blindness is a common result and most frequently occurs in children.

Does vitamin A deficiency result in adverse skin changes?

Dry, rough skin specially in shoulder area is the first symptom. Small bumps near the base of hair follicles known as folliculosis develops.

Does deficiency of vitamin A affects respiratory systems also?

It has always been designated as anti infective agent. Vitamin A deficiency usually lead to bronchial pneumonia. High vitamin A does helps in early recovery in T.B.

What other symptoms develop in vitamin A deficiency?

- Vitamin A deficiency leads to defective formation of enamel layer.
- Loss of taste and smell both occurs in vitamin A deficiency.

What are the signs of vitamin A toxicity?

The symptoms of vitamin A toxicity are many, ranging from headache, drowsiness, nausea, loss of hair, dry skin and diarrhoea.

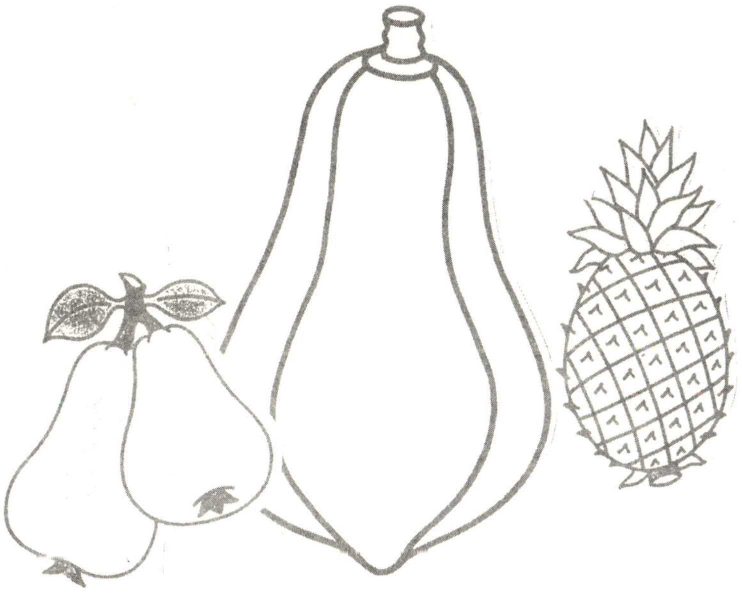

Rapid resorption of bone occurs in adults. To develop symptoms it may take 6-15 months but recovery is rapid and complete on withdrawl of excess intake. Permanent effects of vitamin A toxicity are rare.

VITAMIN E

When was vitamin E discovered?

It was first recognised as a dietary essential in 1922. At that time it was found to be essential for reproduction in rats. Then vitamin E was known as antisterility factor.

What are the chemical forms of vitamin E available?

The term vitamin E is applied to a group of at least light chemical compounds related to d-alpha-tocoferol the most active form of vitamin E in food. Beta and gamma tocoferol is 50% and 10% potent respectively. Alpha tocoferol found in barely is 30% active.

What are the functions of vitamin E?

Vitamin E acts to stabilize PUFA and phospholipids in cell membrane and to protect them from oxidation.

Is vitamin E antioxidant?

By being readily oxidized or using oxygen itself it leaves minimal amount of oxygen for others. Thus fats containing E are less susceptible to oxidation and resulting rancidity. Vitamin A, unsaturated fatty acids and vitamin C in food are similarly protected against destruction.

Is vitamin E helpful in pregnancy too?

Vitamin E may prevent the formation of lipofuscin pigment known as 'ceroid pigment' which accumulates in uterus and may cause fetal death.

What is ceroid pigment?

The accumulation of ceroid pigments characterizes the aging process. But excessive consumption of vitamin E will help.

Does vitamin E helps in cellular respiration?

Vitamin E plays role by which energy from glucose and fatty acids is finally released and water is formed.

Can vitamin E helps in heme synthesis?

Synthesis of heme in iron containing compound which is an essential part of many proteins is dependent on two enzymes whose synthesis is regulated by vitamin E.

What is the role of vitamin E in membrane metabolism?

In deficiency of vitamin E membrane of RBC is weakened. Then membrane can be ruptured. It is caused by oxidation of lipid in membrane.

Is there any relationship between vitamin A & E?

(i) Vitamin E spares vitamin A. (ii) It protects vitamin A from oxidation in gut (iii) it increases absorption of vitamin A (iv) increases storage of vitamin A.

How is vitamins E absorbed?

It requires the presence of bile for absorption. It is best absorbed in presence of fact. At normal levels of intake 40 to 50% of vitamin E is absorbed. As intake increases rate of absorption decreases. Vitamin E is being stored in many tissues of body. Amongst them adipose tissue, muscle and liver are the major sites. This vitamin is excreted in urine or bile.

What is the expected daily requirement of vitamin E?

Previously it was expressed in units I.U. now it is expressed as tocopherol equivalents.

ITE vitamin E = 1.5 I.U. when PUFA content of diet is high requirement of vitamin E also increases. Almost always an increase in PUFA is the result of an increased use of vegetable oils. Since there are also good sources of vitamin E deficiencies of it hardly occurs.

15. I.U. or 10 mg TE or daily requirement will serve the need.

What is the vitamin E oil content of some oil?

Tocopherol content of 100 gm of oils

Oil	Mg/100 gram
Wheat	255
Corn oil	52
Soyabean oil	94
Cotton seed oil	65
Safflower oil	38
Olive oil	12
Coconut oil	4

What are the food sources of vitamin E?

Tocoferol occurs in greatest concentration in vegetable oils. Tocoferol is destroyed in cooking soil but more during freezing.

Fruits and vegetables are relatively poor source of tocopherol but fresh and frozen vegetables retain much more than canned products.

How much vitamin E is available in eatables?

Food	Mg Available
Spinach	2.0
Beef	1.62
Egg	1.42
Butter	1
Tomatoes	0.85
Green peas	0.65
Chicken	0.58
Corn flakes	0.43
Banana	0.42
Carrots	0.21
Orange juice	0.20
Potato	0.056

About 64% of vitamin E comes from oil, 11% from fruits/ vegetables 7% grains. Vitamins E of cereals is destroyed during processing.

What are the effect of vitamin E deficiency?

In human being not much of deficiency signs are known. Blood levels will be lowered down. Anemia may develop.

VITAMIN – D

It has been known as sunshine vitamin because it comes from sun. It cannot be produced by body and some think it is a steroid. It was discovered in 1924 by Mellanby. The existence of provitamin D which could be activated into vitamin D by short uteraviolet rays was discovered in 1922.

How vitamin D is absorbed?

Dietary vitamin D is absorbed primarily in the upper part of small intestine. Once absorbed it is incorporated into small fat particles in chylomicrons and transported in lymphatic system. Bile helps in its absorption.

How vitamin D is excreted?

Most vitamin D is excreted in the bile as a part of bile acid.

What are the functions of vitamin D?

(i) Once active form of vitamin D has been produced it is transported to the intestine, bones and kidneys and helps in çalcification of bone tissue.

(ii) In the bone cell, calcitriol together with parathyroid hormone stimulates release of calcium in blood.

(iii) In the kidneys it increases the amount of calcium and phosphorus reabsorbed of aminoacids in tubules.

What are the units of vitamin D?

It is measured in terms of international units. One I.U. of vitamin D weighs 0.025 mg and 1 mg contains 40,000 I.U.

What is the daily requirement of vitamin D?

As little as 100 I.U. will promote bone development and prevent rickets. Recommended allowance is of 400 I.U. To meet the requirement of 200 I.U. is recommended in pregnancy.

What are the sources of vitamin D?

Exposure to sunlight, fish liver oils and commercial vitamin D preparations are sources of vitamin D. Small amounts are present in egg yolk, liver and fish.

How exposure to sunlight brings about synthesis of vitamin D?

Exposure to sunlight brings about synthesis of vitamin D from the precursor 7 dehydrocholesterol. Sunlight cannot always be dependent upon to supply the body. Because rays are easily strained out by dust, smoke, fog, clothing and window glass. All acts as barrier.

What is hypervitaminosis D?

Tolerance for vitamin D varies widely. 45 mg (18800 I.U.) over a long period may prove toxic to children. Symptoms of toxicity include nausea, vomiting, excessive thirst. There may be renal damage and calcification of soft tissue.

What are the effects of vitamin D deficiency?

Deficiency of vitamin D leads to inadequate absorption of calcium and phosphorus from gastro intestinal tract. It leads to faulty mineralization of bone and tooth.

Does rickets develop due to vitamin D deficiency?

Premature infants are more susceptible. The salient features of rickets are

(i) Soft, fragile bones. Widening of long bones. Enlargement of costochondral junction.

(ii) Pigeon breast, narrowing of pelvis and spinal curvature.

(iii) Delayed closure of fontanelles and bossing of forehead.

(iv) Poorly developed muscles.

(v) Pot belly

(vi) Restlessness and nervous irritability.

What is Tetany?

Tetany is characterized by a low serum calcium i.e. 7.5 mg /100 ml. It results in muscle twitching, cramps, and convulsions. Actually it results from inefficient absorption of calcium and vitamin D.

What is osteomalacia?

It is an adult rickets. Literally it means softening of bones. It occurs when there is lack of vitamin D and calcium.

Features of osteomalacia are –

(i) Bone of legs, spine, thorax and pelvis bends and becomes deformed due to softness.

(ii) There may be generalised pain

(iii) Person may develop spontaneous fractures.

VITAMIN K

When vitamin K was discovered?

It was discovered in 1935 a Koagulation vitamin needed to prevent fatal hemorrhage by Dr. Dam of Copenhagen.

What about the chemistry of vitamin K?

Vitamin K consists of a number of related compounds known as guiones. Menadione is a synthetic compound that is 2-3 times more potent than natural vitamin K.

What are its units of measure?

It is a fat soluble and requires bile for its absorption. Its activity is measured in micrograms by its ability to prevent hemorrhage in chicks.

What about its physiology?

Most of it occurs in upper part of small intestine. This vitamin can also be synthesized by bacteria in lower intestine. 50% of it is derived from plant sources and rest is synthesized by bacteria. New born infant contains minimum of vitamin K so first few days remains critical.

What are the functions of vitamin K?

- It is essential for formation of prothrombin and other clotting proteins by liver.
- It acts as a cofactor for an enzyme in liver
- It is assumed to be required for the synthesis of protein containing Y carboxy glutamic acid.

What is the daily requirement of vitamin K?

Because this vitamin is partly synthesised by intestine not much of it is required from outside. Only 1-2 microgram per kg will be sufficient.

Recommended intake for adults is 70 to 140 mg/day.

What are the food sources of vitamin K?

Dark green leafy vegetables contain more of vitamin K. Alfaalfa is an especially rich source. Average diet provides 0.3 to 0.5 mg/day.

What are the signs of deficiency of vitamin K?

In infants lack of bacteria to synthesize vitamin K, the low stores of vitamin K in infant at birth and low content of milk leads to low prothrombin levels.

WATER SOLUBLE VITAMINS

Water soluble vitamins are considered essential and plays a specific role in body metabolism. Two main vitamins are B-complex and vitamin C.

VITAMIN C

What is the history of vitamin C?

Description of vitamin C can be found in 1500 BC in writings of Hippocrates in 400 BC. In 1906 it was recognised as deficiency disease. In 1932 King and Waugh isolated it from lemon juice. Spaniards landing after long sea voyages in California in 1602, 1603 and again in 1769 lost many of their members due to scurvy.

What are the chemical properties of vitamin C?

Chemically ascorbic acid is simple 6 carbon compound related to monosaccharides. In solution it is stable but is easily destroyed on exposure to air, light, alkali and heat in presence of copper and iron.

Is there synthetic ascorbic acid too?

Synthetic ascorbic acid is used to enrich food products and as nutrient supplement. It is as good as natural ascorbic acid.

How synthesis of vitamin C takes place?

Most animals can synthesize it from glucose and therefore need no dietary supply of it. It takes place in liver cells.

In plants ascorbic acid is accumulated during the ripening process.

What are the functions of Ascorbic acid?

In contrast to most water soluble vitamins it has no clear cut role as a catalyst nor it is a part of enzyme.

Does vitamin C helps in collagen formation?

It forms collagen by fibroblasts in connective tissue. Collagen is a major component of skin, cartilage, teeth and scar tissue. In the absence of ascorbic acid collagen cannot be found and tropo-collagen is degraded into its component aminoacid.

Failure in collagen synthesis also shows up as small pinpoint hemorrhages resulting from weakness of capillaries and in fibres that join the cells together. The matrix which makes up 1/5th of bone shaft is collagen only.

Is vitamin C helpful in dentin formation?

The dentin layer arising from a group of cells known as odontoblasts does not form normally in the absence of vitamin C due to the failure of producing a matrix.

Does it help in synthesis of neurotransmitters?

(i) Two transmitters in brain are needed to transfer nerve impulses from one cell to another. These function in presence of vitamin C only.

(ii) Vitamin C is needed to convert tyrosine and tryptophane to the precursor of neurotransmitter norepinephrine and serotonin which regulates blood pressure.

Does vitamin C helps in utilization of iron and calcium?

For absorption of iron from intestine vitamin C is required. It also helps in transfer of transferrin to ferritin in which form iron is stored.

Vitamin C helps in absorption of calcium by creating an acid medium in stomach.

Similarly the conversion of inactive form of folic acid to active form, the cytrovorum factor is catalysed by ascorbic acid.

What are other functions of vitamin C?

(i) Large does of vitamin C have been beneficial to low environmental temperatures.

(ii) It helps in early healing of wounds.

(iii) It is useful in preventing atherosclerosis.

(iv) It helps adrenals in the synthesis of steroid hormone nor – epinephrine.

How vitamin C is being absorbed?

It is absorbed in upper part of intestine by simple diffusion and is circulated in blood. In low doses absorption is 90% but absorption decreases as doses increase.

The total pool of ascorbic acid has been estimated to be 1500 mg on an intake of 100 mg daily.

How vitamin C is excreted?

It is excreted primarily in urine. Although this vitamin is reabsorbed while passing through kidney to maintain level of 1.2 to 1.4 mg/100 ml. Once body level of 1500 mg is reached rest is lost in urine.

What is the daily requirement of vitamin C?

Daily requirement of 50 mg will meet the requirement. Infants on mother's milk should receive more.

What will happen is consumed much more than requirement?

Then ascorbic acid will be excreted unchanged. More than that can contribute to the formation of kidney stones from accumulated oxalic acid.

What will be the effect of refrigeration?

Storing of vegetables at refrigerator temperature in high humidity with a little air movement will reduce vitamin C. Then it depends on vegetable to vegetable. Losses of 88% ascorbic acid in green beans and none in broccoli after 6 days at 2.2^{0}C is noted.

What is the effect of cooking on vitamin C?

Heat reduces vitamin C content. If processing is done in absence of air, losses will be much lower. If you want to have full content of vitamin C then you have to consume in raw state. The amount of water used in cooking has a greater effect on losses than does the total cooking. Steaming was better than boiling. Microwave cooking causes less destruction of vitamin C.

What are the important food sources of vitamin C?

Dietary sources of vitamin C

Food	Mg/100 gm	Food	Mg/100
Guava	200-300	Citrons fruits	30-63
Lime	63	Capsicum	180
Orange	30	Cabbage	124
Tomato	27	Amla	600
Spinach	28	Potato	17
Cholai	99	Onion	11

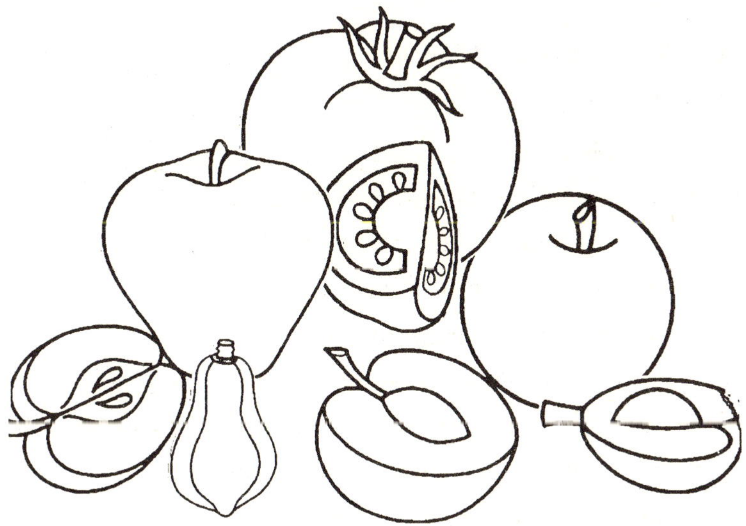

What is the commercial use of vitamin C?

It is used as a preservative in jams and jellies, a colour stabilizer in fruit cocktail. It is a dough conditioner in white flour, an acidulant in frozen deserts and in wine and beer it prevents darkening of colour and maintains flavour.

What are the deficiency signs of vitamin 'C'?

Infants only on milk diet may develop anorexia, growth failure, tenderness of hip and anemia. Onset is rapid. Delayed and incomplete wound healing is a frequent manifestation.

How excessive consumption of vitamin C affects vitamin B_{12}.

It may destruct vitamin B_{12} a decrease in copper absorption, an, increase in plasma cholesterol, interference with anticoagulants, destruction of RBCS and in rare cases reproductive failure.

VITAMIN B-COMPLEX

THIAMINE

When thiamine was discovered?

It was discovered by Willians in 1936. Germans found it in rice bran to treat 'Beri Beri' In 1890 a Dutch physician had treated polyneuritis in chickens with it.

What are the chemical properties of B_1?

It is a white crystalline substance soluble in water. It is easily destroyed by heat or oxidation. It has antineuritic factor indicative of its role in preventing systems involving nerves.

What are the function of thiamine?

- It acts in carbohydrate metabolism.

- It acts in transmission of high frequency impulses at the nerve synapse through the production or release of neurotransmitter acetylcholine.
- It plays role in conversion of aminoacid tryptophan to niacin.

How thiamine is being absorbed?

Absorption occurs in duodenum 2.5 to 5mg daily. Large amounts are absorbed by passive effusion.

A substance in onion oil and garlic oil allin combines with thiamine to form allin thiamine a form in which thiamine is radily absorbed.

Body contains 30-70 mg of thiamine. Half is distributed in muscles excess of thiamine is excreted in urine.

What is the daily requirement of thiamine?

Its need is dependent on calorie requirement. Increased carbohydrate need increases the need of thiamine. In pregnancy and old age need increases. Increased consumption of alcohol also increases its demand. Fat protects thiamine from loss or destruction in body. Recommend daily in take is 0.4 mg / 1000 Kcal or about 1.2 mg in adult man.

Limited amount may be synthesized by microorganism in G.I.track.

What are the rich sources of thiamine?

Important sources are dried yeast, unmilled cereals and pulses, oil seeds specially ground nuts. In cereals it is richly available in outer layer hence machine milled rice is a poor source.

Thiamine content mg / 100gm

Food	mg%	Food	mg%
Rice home pounded	0.21	Milk Cow	0.05
Rice milled	0.6	Egg hen	0.10
Almonds	0.24	Mutton	0.18
Groundnut	0.90	Liver sheep	0.36
Wheat whole	0.45		

Richest sources of vitamin are pork preparations.

The use of bread products provide enough thiamine to ensure an adequate intake of diets.

How thiamine is lost?

- Loss of solution – water will reach out a product (thiamine) in proportion to the amount of water available, As much as 18% of thiamine is lost in preparation of rice.
- Loss from heat – Thiamine is destroyed by temperatures above 100°c. Higher the heat greater the loss.
- Loss from oxidation – Cooking procedures that increase the amount of oxygen in contact with the food. In moist heat speed of destruction is more.
- Loss from alkali – The destruction is greatest in presence of alkali i.e baking soda.
- Loss from irradiation – Thiamine is virtually destroyed by irradiation procedures used in food preservation.

What are the deficiency signs of thiamine?

It may result from failure of absorption due to folic acid deficiency or there may be a lack of supply or inability of tissues to accumulate it. Symptoms of deficiency will be:-

- Loss of appetite – Deficiency of thiamine has clearly demonstrated loss of appetite accompanied with vomiting.
- Decreased muscle tone – Elasticity of tone of wall of lower G.I.T drops in thiamine deficiency. Colon is distended and constipation will result.
- Depression – Mental depression and confusion are relieved by administration of sufficient thiamine in the dose of 1.4 mg daily for months.
- Neurological changes – It causes weakness in sixth cranial nerve. Levels of thiamine can be reduced to 50% of niacin content. When it remains only 30% gait may become slow and unsteady and at 20% severe disturbance of posture and equilibrium occurs. Neuromuscular coordination is affected in persons on low thiamine intake.

What is Beri Beri?

In china it was known before 2600BC. But the cause of beri beri was not identified. The practice of repeatedly washing and cooking looses thiamine. It is more common in breast fed children. Human milk contains 50% thiamine than cow's milk.

What are the symptoms of Beri Beri in infants?

Symptoms develop very fast and child develops cyanosis. Heart beat fastens and cry changes from loud piercing one to a thin, weak, almost inaudible one. Some may develop vomiting and convulsions. Once thiamine is made available symptoms disappears.

How many types of Beri Beri are there?

There are two types of Beri Beri

i. Dry Beri Beri

ii. Wet beri Beri

What are the Symptoms of dry beri beri?

- In dry beri beri there develops gradual loss of body tissue.
- Patient becomes thin and emaciated.
- Swelling develops from foot and gradually progresses upwards.
- Heart size may be increased .
- Difficulty in walking.
- Wrist / ankle drop.

What are the symptoms of wet Beri beri?

- Gradually loss of body weight occurs.
- Numbness in arms & legs.
- Irritability
- Vague uneasiness.
- Disorderly thinking

It is more common where polished rice is eaten.

RIBOFLAVIN

What is Riboflavin?

It is also known as vitamin B_2.It is known for growth and tissue repair. In 1952 it become evident that active factor was composed of a protein plus a pigment the flavin.

What are the chemical properties of riboflavin?

It is relatively an stable vitamin. It is resistant to heat, acid and oxidation. But it is unstable in presence of alkali and light. It is less soluble in water so some losses occur when smaller pieces cut and boiled in large amount of water.

What are the functions of riboflavin?

- It is part of several enzymes and coenzymes.
- It is needed to release energy from glucose and fatty acids with in the cell mitochondrion.
- It is also involved in conversion of folic acid to its coenzyme and their storage in body.

How riboflavin is being absorbed?

Its absorption takes place in upper portion of G.I.Tract. 60% riboflavin is absorbed when taken with meals.

How riboflavin is excreted?

It is excreted primarily in the urine. A little is excreted in stool too.Very little riboflavin is absorbed in body.

What are the daily requirements of riboflavin?

For all ages 0.6mg of riboflavin per 1000kcal with a minimum of 1.2mg is recommended. During pregnancy 0.3mg daily is needed and during lactation 0.5mg.

What are the food sources of riboflavin?

It is widely distributed in animals and vegetables. About 90% of vitamin is retained in fruits and vegetable. Milk makes a significant contribution.

Palm Juice 'Neera' is a rich source of it . A diet high in fat and protein results in decreased synthesis of it in intestines while diet high in starch, lactose and cellulose increases its synthesis.

What are the deficiency signs of riboflavin?

- Early symptom is cheilosis i.e cracks appear at the corners of mouth.

- Tongue becomes smooth and becomes purplish red colour i.e glossitis.
- Skin becomes dry and scaly.
- Retardation of growth occurs.
- Reproduction capacity is reduced.

NIACIN

What is niacin?

It is known as nicotinic acid and rarely as B_3. In 1987 it was known as antipellagra factor. Pellagra is prevalent in maize eaters.

What are chemical properties of it?

It is extremely stable to heat, acid, alkali or light. Little is lost during cooking. It is active as the amide nicotinamide.

What is the relationship between tryptophan and niacin?

Tryptophan is also effective in curing pellagra. So deficiency alone of niacin may produce pellagra. The conversion of tryptophan to niacin requires the presence of thiamine, pyridoxin and riboflavin.

What are the functions of niacin?

- It is required in the release of energy from fats, proteins and carbohydrates.
- It is involved in the synthesis of protein.

How riboflavin is being utilized?

Naicin is readily absorbed and is stored to a limited extent. About 2/3rd of niacin is metabolized from tryptophan.

What is the requirement of niacin?

Daily requirement is 4.4 niacin equivalent for 1000 calories. Total if one takes 13NE will serve the purpose.

In addition to gastro intestinal symptoms , unusual nervousness, recurring increased uric acid secretion and glucose intolerance develop.

PYRIDOXINE

It is known as Vitamin B_6 also. In 1934 Gyorgy suggested the name pyridoxine.

What are its functions?

- It acts as a coenzyme for many biological reactions.
- It is necessary in both synthesis and catabolism of aminoacids.
- Pyridoxal phosphate plays a role in hemoglobin synthesis.
- It is essential for the production of antibodies.

What is the daily requirement of it?

Daily-recommended dose is 2mg per day. Treatment with certain drug e.g. INH, hydralazine and oral contraceptive may cause deficiency of this vitamin

What are the rich sources of vitamin?

Pyridoxin content micro gm / 100gm

Food	µgm	Food	µgm
Chicken	683	Beans	150
Banana	510	Potatoes	51
Ham	400	Cheese	80
Egg yolk	300	Milk	40
Cabbage	160	Orange Juice	28

It is found widely distributed in natrure. In plants it occurs as pyridoxine.

Amongst the richest are chicken fish, liver, whole grains, cereals , and egg yolk. Citrous fruit milk cheese are poor source.

Freezing of vegetables causes 25% loss and milling of cereals cuases about 90% of original values.

What are its deficiencies signs in infant?

The infant shows nervous irritability and convulsive seizures. Other related symptoms are anemia, vomiting, weakness, abdominal pain and ataxia.

PANTOTHENIC ACID

It is known as vitamin B_3. It is yellow, viscous oil.

What are its chemical properties?

It is water soluble and readily destroyed by heat. It unites with a sulphur containing, amino acid alanine. Co-enzyme A is the form in which most pantothenic acid is found.

What are its functions?

- Pantothenic acid participates release of energy from all three fat, carbohydrate and protein.
- It provides acetyl groups for the formation of acetylcholine needed in the transmission of nerve impulses.
- It helps in detoxification of drugs.
- It is essential for the formation of porphyrin.
- It stimulates anti body response.
- It stimulates synthesis of cholesterol.

What is the daily requirement?

Its daily requirement is 5 to 10mg or 10 times more requirement of thiamine. Except for period of stress such as pregnancy most

Fruits and vegetables make a much more important contribution. Beans, Spinach, lemons, are good sources of it.

Does food processing has any effect on folic acid?

Losses of folic acid in processing and cooking may range as high as 50-90%High temperature and large volumes of water are harmful. Free folacin activity of frozen dinners on reheating losses. Folic acid by 22% exposes to light reduces its quality.

What are the deficiency signs of Folic acid?

Deficiency of it may result due to

- Inadequate intake
- Impaired absorption
- Excessive demands
- Increased losses
- Metabolic derangements

It results in megaloblastic anemia.

What are the clinical use of folic acid?

It is effective in treating nutritional megaloblastic anemia.

It relieves symptoms of tropical sprue, glossitis and gastro intestinal disturbance.

What are toxicity signs of folic acid?

There appears to be no toxic reactions to folic acid. Even if 15mg is taken for 1 month no adverse effect will develop. Large amounts may interfere with the action of drugs such as anticonvulsants.

COBALAMIN

Till 1926 pernicious anemia was known as a fatal disease. Large doses of liver were found effective. It is known as vitamin B_{12}.

What is the chemical composition of it?

Commercial vitamin B_{12} is primarily cyanocobalamin obtained by bacterial synthesis. Since it contains cobalt it has B_{12} activity. Crystals are bright red due to which it was known as red vitamin.

What are the functions of B_{12}?

- It is necessary for normal growth.
- It is required for normal blood formation.
- It maintains working nervous systems.
- It is necessary for the release of folic acid from methyl folate.

How vitamin B_{12} is absorbed?

As food passes through the digestive tract acid of gastric juice and pancreatic juice causes release of vitamin B_{12} from food. Most of elderly people who no longer secrete gastric acid are unable to absorb B_{12} from food.

How vitamin B_{12} is metabolized?

Once cobalamine is absorbed it passes to blood stream. Here it was bound to a transport protein known as transcobolamin. In this form only it circulates to various tissues.

About 2% of vitamin B12 is excreated in bile. Excess is stored in liver. Liver is able to store 2000 microgram sufficient to last for 6 years.

What is the requirement of vitamin B_{12}?

Daily requirement is 0.6 to 1.0 microgram. Fetus draws about 0.3 microgram of it from mother. Which has to be supplemented to mother.

What are the food sources of vitamin B_{12}?

It is present only in animals and fruits / vegetables contain only

Minerals

Ninety six percent of body weight is made up of carbon hydrogen and oxygen,proteins and water. Remaining 4% i.e. about 2.5kg is made up of 60 elements out of it 21 have been proved essential for body.

How to classify elements?

i. Macronutrients are

Calcium	1.5 – 2.2 % of body weight
Phosphorus	0.8 – 1.2 % of body weight
Potassium	0.35 % of body weight
Sodium	0.15 % of body weight
Chlorine	0.15 % of body weight
Magnesium	0.05 % of body weight

ii. Micronutrients are

Iron	0.004% of body weight
Zinc	0.002% of body weight
Selenium	0.0003% of body weight
Mangnese	0.0002% of body weight
Copper	0.00015% of body weight
Iodine	0.0004% of body weight

CALCIUM

In the adult body between 1.5% and 2% of weight is calcium.

What are the factors helping in absorption of calcium?

When vitamin D is present calcium is absorbed throughout a greater part of intestine.

How acidity affects absorption of calcium?

Calcium is soluble in acid than in alkaline medium. In old age hydrochloric content of stomach decreases so is calcium absorption.

Does lactose also helps in absorption of calcium?

Yes presence of disaccharide and lactose increases absorption from 15% to 50%. Lactose facilitates the passive diffusion of calcium into blood .

What should be the calcium / phosphorus ratio?

Two parts of calcium and 1-2 parts of phosphorus promotes the highest level of absorption. For infant ratio of 1.3:1 is advised.

Does absorption of calcium depends on the need of the body?

Yes, the extent to which calcium is absorbed may be influenced by the body's need for calcium. During pregnancy, lactation and adolescence needs are greatest and 50% of calcium is being absorbed.

Does oxalic acid decreases the absorption of calcium?

Oxalic acid combines with calcium to form insoluble calcium oxalate from which calcium cannot be released for its absorption. But there is no evidence that oxalic acid of spinach will interfere in absorption of calcium of milk.

Does phytic acid lowers down the absorption of calcium?

Phytic acid lowers the utilization of calcium by binding it in an insoluble complex.

Is protein and high fat consumption helps in calcium absorption?

It is assumed that high protein diet must be improving absorption of calcium. While high fat diets, the formation of insoluble soaps of fatty acids and calcium results in fatty stools and a reduction in calcium absorption . At least long chain fatty acids depress calcium absorption.

Will increased gastrointestinal motility affect on the absorption of calcium?

Any cause which increases intestinal motility decreases absorption of calcium. Luxatives and foods high in bulk may have this effect.

How lack of exercise affects its absorption?

Bed ridden persons and who do not exercise experience a loss of 0.5% of total stores every month and develops a reduced ability to replace it.

How calcium is metabolized?

Once calcium is absorbed in intestine it is transported to blood plasma and then to tissues. From there cells absorb whatever the calcium is needed. As blood plasma is filtered through kidneys 99% of calcium is reabsorbed and 1% is excreted in urine.

Most of the absorbed calcium is used in the calcification of bones to give strength. Deposition of calcium in bone is helped by vitamin D and phosphatase .

About 1/3rd of calcium is available in blood 9 to 11mg/dl.

What is the role of parathyroid in absorption of calcium?

The parathyroid gland has a major role in maintaining blood calcium level. When calcium levels fall below 7mg /dl parathyroid secretes a parathyroid hormone. With in minutes kidneys are

Rich sources of calcium gm/100gm.

Food	gm / 100gm	Food	gm /100gm
Milk	0.12	Carrot	0.34
Milk buffalo	0.21	Fish dried	1.8
Cheese	0.79	Sitaphal	0.8
Blackgram	0.20	Mint	0.20

Eggshell contains 2gms of calcium.

What will happen if more calcium is being consumed?

High intake would not result in kidney stones or will not lead to deposition of calcium in other soft tissues. Soft tissue deposition is more likely due to low magnesium than of high calcium.

High intake of calcium may have depressing effect on utilization of phosphorus, copper, iodine, zinc, magnesium and iron.

What is osteoporosis?

It is generally found in females especially after menopause resulting in susceptibility of fractures and low backache. Women looses as much as 9%of their compact bone. It is attributed as decrease in bone mass due to long standing dietary inadequacy and poor absorption of calcium.

A diet high in calcium 1.5gm daily and 50mg/day of sodium fluoride and with adequate vitamin D proves useful in prevention of osteoporosis.

What is osteomalacia?

It generally develops in those women who wear 'burkas', live in areas of low sunshine, whose diets are low in calcium. Who are on anticonvulsant drugs, multipara and feed their children for long.

Most such cases respond to vitamin D therapy. There may also be low phosphorus levels.

What is hypercalcemia?

It is reported in infants as the result of high intakes of vitamin D or when phosphorus to calcium ratio is very high. Sometime whole milk formulas interfere with the absorption of calcium. Best is to reduce vitamin D intake rather than reducing calcium level.

What do you understand by calcium rigor?

When calcium level falls low there is change in stimulation of nerve cells which result in increased excitability of nerve and spasmodic and uncontrolled contraction of muscle tissue known as tetany. When calcium rises above particular level the muscle fibres enter a stage of tonic contraction known as calcium rigor.

How higher intake of phosphorus affects calcium level?

High phosphorus intakes lead to a loss of calcium as a result of parathyroid horomone secretion which causes bone resorption . Ratio of phosphorus to calcium should remain 2:1.

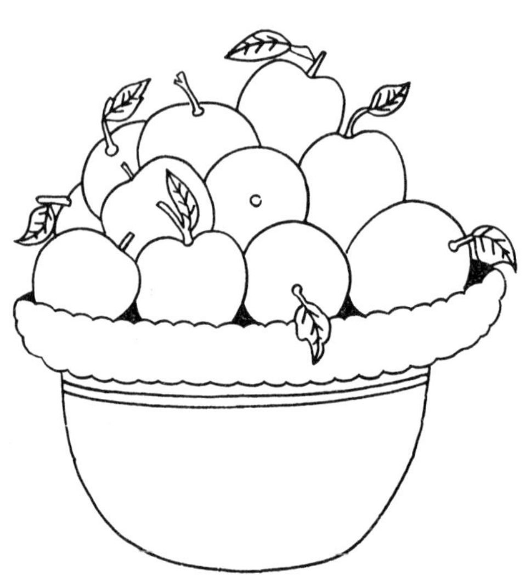

PHOSPHORUS

1% of body weight is phosphorus so it is known as macronutrient. Body contains about 12gm of phosphorus per kg .of fat free tissue. Of this 85% is in the form of insoluble calcium phosphate. It gives rigidity and strength to bones .

How phosphorus helps in regulation of energy?

It is necessary for controlled release of energy from combustion of carbohydrate, fat and protein. Energy is stored when a third phosphate molecule is attached to ADP to ATP.

Does phosphorus helps in absorption of nutrients?

Fats which are insoluble in water are transported in blood as phospholipids. When glycogen is released from the liver or muscle storage it is released as phosphorylated glucose. Phosphorylation occurs in absorption from the intestine.

Can phosphorus help in regulation of acid base balance?

Because phosphorus can combine with additional hydrogen ions, it becomes an important buffer to prevent a change in the acidity of body fluids .

How phosphorus helps in calcification of bone and teeth?

Calcification process involves the fixation of phosphate to the matrix. It is the deficiency of phosphate and not calcium which hampers bone formation.

Is phosphorus part of body compounds?

Since all enzymes are proteins and many proteins contain phosphorus tells its importance. Phosphate is an integral part of nucleic acids DNA and RNA both of which are essential for bone formation .

How phosphorus is absorbed and metabolized?

The amount of phosphorus absorbed varies inversely with the amount of magnesium, iron and other elements. Only 70% dietary phosphorus is absorbed. Phytic acid is only 50% absorbed. Parathyroid hormone and vitamin D regulates phosphorus /calcium ratio.

What are the rich sources of phosphorus?

Generally foods rich in protein are also rich in phosphorus. Meat, fish, poultry cereals and eggs are primary source of phosphorus in average diet.

Phosphorus mg/100gm.

Food	mg / 100gm	Food	mg / 100gm
Cheese	512	Peas	116
Peanuts	401	Beans	67
Whole Wheat	228	Rice cooked	28
Eggs	180		

What is its daily requirement?

Daily requirement is of 800mg /day. 2/3 of it is required before 6 months of age.

What are the probable signs of deficiency of phosphorus?

Deficiency of it generally does not occur but who consumes lot of antacids absorption of phosphorus may suffer, from it fatigue, loss of appetite and demineralization of result.

MAGNESIUM

Magnesium is known since 1859. In plant it is essential occurring predominantly with in cell. Whole body contains 21 to 28 gm. Of which 60% is present in bone.Remaining 40%

is in muscle and tissues. It is absorbed primarily in small intestine. Excretion of it is through kidney.

What are functions of magnesium?

- It acts as catalyst to several hundred biological reactions.
- Magnesium influences protein synthesis.
- It helps in nerve conduction.
- It acts and allows muscle contraction.
- It increases the stability of calcium in tooth enamel.
- It helps in secretion of thyroxin.

What are the signs of deficiency?

- When person is on starvation signs of its deficiency appears.
- There may be low magnesium tetany similar to that when blood calcium level falls.
- There may be convulsive seizures.
- Alcohol increases the rate of magnesium excretion.
- There may be vasodilation.

What is the daily requirement?

Age	Requirement mg
1-10 years	150-250
11-14 years	300-350
15-18 years	300-400
Adult man	350
Adult woman	300
Pregnancy / Lactation	450

What are the food sources?

Vegetables are the best source followed by legumes, seafood, nuts, cereals and dairy products. Rice and soyabean are very rich source.

SODIUM

In 1937 sodium as a dietary supplement was established. It is a monovalent positively charged ion. 10% is present in cells, 40% sodium is found in the skeleton bound in surface of bone crystals. Rest is in body fluids.

What are the functions of sodium?

- It accounts for most of the osmotic pressure.
- Sodium accounts for 90% of the alkalinity of extracellular fluids and maintains body neutrality.
- Contraction of muscles involves a temporary exchange of sodium and potassium in the contracting muscle cell.
- Sodium is essential for absorption of glucose.

What is the daily requirement of sodium?

Requirement of sodium is determined by the needs for growth, loses of sweat and other secretions.Daily requirement of 3 to 7gm is sufficient.

Safe of sodium intake is

Age Group	Mg / day of sodium
4-6 years	450 – 1300
7-10 years	600 – 1800
11 years	900 – 2700
Adults	1100 – 3300

What are the food sources of sodium?

It is more prevalent in nonvegetarian diet than in plants.

Sodium content of foods mg / 100gm

Food	Mg / 100mg
Apples	1
Sweet potato	16
Carrots	47
Milk	50
Egg	118
Tomato	200
Cheese	404
Cornflakes	914
Cheese	1310

How sodium is being absorbed?

Small portion is absorbed in stomach but most of it is absorbed in small intestines. About 1gm of it is lost in perspiration.

Is sodium restricted diet helpful in certain diseases?

Yes, in hypertension and kidney disorders it is considered important to restrict sodium intake. Degree of restriction varies with severity of disease.

For a strict limitation to 200mg it is necessary to choose foods low in sodium.

POTASSIUM

It is a positively charged ion similar to sodium. It is concentrated inside the cell rather than extracellular fluid. Ratio of sodium to potassium in cell is 1:10 while in extracellular fluid is 28:1. Body contains 250gm of potassium in body and most of it is in cell.

What are the functions of potassium?

- It acts as a catalysts in releasing energy.
- It helps in glycogen and protein synthesis.
- It maintains osmotic pressure and regulation of fluid balance.
- It maintains acid base balance.
- It helps in transmission of nerve impulses.
- It helps in relaxation of muscles.

What are the signs of potassium deficiency?

Infants suffering from diarrhoea may suffer from it. Vomiting, use of diuretics, severe protein calorie malnutrition may lead it. Symptoms include weakness, poor intestinal tones and weakness of respiratory muscles.

What is the daily requirement?

Estimated requirement is 2 to 6gm / daily or 0.8 to 1.5gm / 1000 calories. Being freely distributed in most eatables deficiency of it hardly occurs.

What are it rich food sources?

3000 – 500 mg	1000 – 300 mg/100gm	Less than 100mg
Liver	Grapses	Egg
Banana	Orange	Bread
Potatos	Apple	Cereals
Peanut butter	Cabbage	Cheese
	Carrots	
	Tomatoes	
	Cheese	
	Chicken	

Because of antagostic relationship between sodium and potassium, excess intake of sodium result in lower absorption of it. Magnesium deficiency also leads to decreased retention of potassium.

CHLORINE

Body contain 0.15% of body weight. In high concentration it is present in G.F.S and gastrointestinal tract. Muscle and nerve tissues are low in chlorine content.

What are the functions of chlorine?

- As a part of hydrochloric acid it maintains the normal acidity.
- It maintains acid base balance.
- Human milk contains more chloride than sodium sufficient to maintain a ratio of 2:1.

How it is excreted?

It is excreted in urine but kidney is efficient in reabsorbing chlorine when dietary intake is low.

SULPHUR

It represents 0.25% of body weight and is present in every cell. It is concentrated in cytoplasm. Higher concentration is found in hair, skin and nails.

What are the functions of sulphur?

- It plays role in formation of blood clot.
- It is a part of at least 4-vitamin thiamine, pantothenic acid, biotin and liopid acid.
- It acts as a coenzyme necessary to activate several enzymes.
- It is necessary for collagen synthesis.

IRON

Iron was identified in 1713. It constitute 0.004% of body weight. Total iron content is 8 to 5 gm.

How iron is distributed in body?

Mostly it is present in blood. Every living cell also contains it. Majority of it is present in hemoglobin molecule of RBC and small portion is part of myoglobin.

About 70% iron is functional iron rest of 30% is present in spleen.

Distribution of iron

	Total %	Adults mg.
Hemoglobin	60 – 75%	2100
Myoglobin	3	100
Spleen / bone marrow	0 – 30	1000
Tissue iron	5 – 15	350
Transferrin	1	4
Serum Ferritin	1	0.3
Total		3554.3

Is iron a carrier of oxygen and carbon dioxide?

It is a basic biochemical role of iron to transfer O_2 and CO_2 from one tissue to another. It is also a part of many enzymes.

Does it help in blood formation?

It forms hemoglobin which is an essential component of RBCs. Hence an iron containing protein is synthesized in the presence of B_6. Adult male has 15 gram of hemoglobin per 100 ml.

What are the other functions of iron?

Other functions include.

- Catalysing the conversion of beta-carotene.
- Precursor of vitamin A to vitamin A.
- Synthesis of purines.
- Removal of lipids from blood
- Collagen synthesis.
- Detoxification of drugs.

How much is the loss of iron daily?

Before absorption iron must be separated from its organic complex and any ferric iron should be changed to ferrous iron. For it gastric HCL or vitamin C is required. Absorption occurs primarily in the upper part of small intestine usually the duodenum.

What are the factors affecting absorption of iron?

Person with normal hemoglobin level absorbs from 2 to 10% dietary iron. In anemia absorption may go upto 30%. Progressive absorption is noted in later half of pregnancy.

What type of iron is more beneficial?

Ferrous iron is better absorbed than ferric one. Vitamin C of fruits helps in changing ferric to ferrous acid.

How much iron is being absorbed?

Only 5% of iron of most vegetable foods is absorbed such as from rice, corn, spinach where as 20% of meat and 10% of fish iron is being absorbed. The consumtion of meat in conjunction with vegetable increases the absorption of iron 2 – 3 folds.

What is the effect of bulk in diet?

Higher fiber and higher cellulose diet depresses iron absorption. Green leafy vegetable iron is being absorbed only 1 – 2%. Hence iron capsules must be taken before meals to avoid interference in absorption. Single large dose of iron is being absorbed less.

What other factors are responsible for iron absorption?

- Phytic acid combines with iron to form an insoluble iron complex which body cannot absorb.
- Excessive phosphorus also inhibit iron absorption .
- Excessive loss of fat in stool reduces iron absorption.
- High altitude increases iron absorption.

How much iron is lost in blood donation?

0.5 liter of iron represent loss of 250mg of iron which must be replaced. The blood volume and cell number will return to normal soon. To replace the amount of iron i.e. 0.7mg will take one year.

Does need of iron increases during growing period?

Due to increase in blood volume during growth will require more of RBCs and hemoglobin. 4.5 mg of iron storage is to be increased from 1 year to 20 years.

What is the daily requirement of iron?

Adult male should get 0.7 to 1 mg of iron to replace body losses and female 1 to 1.2mg daily. So requirement may vary from 10 to 20mg daily

Daily requirement of iron:

Group	mg/day
Adult men / Women	20
Menstruating women	30
Pregnancy	40
Lactation	30
Adolescent girls	35
Adolescent boys	25
Children	15 – 20
Infants	1.0 mg/kg

What is the requirement of iron in pregnancy?

300mg of iron is needed for the fetus, 70mg of iron for placenta and 500mg for synthesis of hemoglobin.

Fetus accumulates 0.5mg/day in first trimester but it increases to 3 to 4 mg day in last 2 trimesters.

What about lactation and iron need?

Human milk contains 0.2μg/ml and is a poor source of iron. The amount of iron is not affected by mothers diet. Since only 0.5 to 1mg is transferred to milk no extra iron is to be consumed. But during pregnancy and delivery some iron is lost so extra consumption of 3 to 6mg daily may be helpful.

Do infants and children require more iron?

The reserve of iron in liver is sufficient for 3 to 6 months. The high hemoglobin level of new born infant drop rapidly to 12gm at 4 to 6 months of age. Infants over 3 months of age should be provided iron drops.

What are the rich iron sources of food?

Liver, Spinach, beans, molasses, jaggery are rich sources of it.

Iron content mg / 100gm

Food	Iron	Food	Iron
Bengal gram	8.8	Bitter guard	9.4
Peas dry	4.4	Jaggery	11.4
Soya bean	11.3	Gingely	10.8
Egg	2.1	Mint	15.6
Mutton	2.5	Spinach	5.0

Meat and citrus fruits enhance iron absorption. Fruits and vegetables are fairly good a source of iron but often due to excessive cellulose iron is not being absorbed. Canned fruits, vegetables cooked in milk products have extra iron. Milk products are poor source of iron.

What is the effect of cooking on iron content?

Loss of iron is in excessive water, which is discarded, and removal of peelings with loss of iron concentrated near the skin. Hence cooking of large pieces of food, cooking with skins on and use of simmering than boiling water will reduce iron loss. Steamed vegetables have more iron.

Can iron be fortified?

For fortification only those food be selected which are consumed in adequate quantity by most of population. Food should remain stable and palatable for long period of time.

What happens in iron deficiency?

Body is very efficient in using iron. Chances of developing iron deficiency are during growth of child, trauma- bleeding or in female who have delivered frequently at short intervals.

Anemia is a condition, which results due to iron deficiency. It can be diagnosed by estimating hemoglobin level.

What is nutritional anemia?

It is caused by absence of any dietary essential involved in hemoglobin formation or by poor absorption. It is due to lack of dietary iron or high quality protein. It is more common in adolescent girls when the growth demands and menstrual losses are difficult to meet.

Infants after 3 months of age on breast formulas should be given iron + Vitamin C drops.

What happens if iron becomes in excess?

Excess of iron may accumulate in normal storage site, liver, and spleen and condition is known as hemosiderosis.

While in hemochromatosis iron is stored in those tissues which generally don't store iron.

IODINE

How is iodine distributed?

In whole body iodine quantity is only 15 to 23mg. 70 to 80% lies in thyroid gland. Rest remains in salivary, mammary or gastric glands and kidneys.

How iodine is absorbed?

Absorption of it takes 3 hours and takes place in gastrointestinal tract, specially in small intestine. Once aborbed it appears in blood. About 30% is absorbed in thyroid and rest is taken up by kidneys to excrete.

What is the function of thyroid?

- It regulates the growth and development of organisms and its metabolism.
- It helps in conversion of carotene to vitamin A.
- It helps in synthesis of protein.
- It helps in absorption of carbohydrate.

What is the daily requirement of it?

Food and water both provide iodine in diet. An iodine content of less than 2μg/l is associated with iodine deficiency. Daily intake of 150μgm is sufficient for an adult.

What are the good food sources of Iodine?

Sea food are the richest sources of it. Salt water fish contains 300 to 3000 microgram of iodine/kg of flash, while fresh water fish contains 20 – 40 μgm (microgram).

Sea salt is not a good source of iodine because iodine voltalizes during drying.

Iodine content in microgram / 100gm

Food	Iodine	Food	Iodine
Apple	1.6	Milk	3.5
Bread	5.8	Pork	4.5
Cabbage	5.2	Potatoes	4.5
Cheese	5.1		
Egg	9.3		

What happens in case of iodine deficiency?

It results in iodine goiter characterized by swelling in neck due to enlargement of thyroid gland. It enlarges because it tries to compensate for lack of iodine

Goiter is a painless condition. Due to pressure it may result in difficulty in breathing.

What is cretinism?

It is seen in children born to mothers who have a limited iodine intake during adolescence and pregnancy. These children are dwarf, mentally retarded, with thick, dry and pasty skin with bulging abdomen. If treated well symptoms may reverse.

What is myxoedema?

Adults suffer from it due to deficiency of iodine. These will have sparsy, coarse, yellowish skin with poor tolerance to cold. These people suffer from low, husky voice.

What happens in hyperthyroidism?

In hyperthyroidism basal metabolic rate is elevated by 100% above normal. Persons develop nervousness, weight loss, increased appetite and intolerance to heat. He develops hand tremors and protruding eyeballs.

ZINC

It is an element present at 50ppm in earth crusts and 23ppm in plants. In 1961 evidence of deficiency showed retarded growth and delayed sexual maturity.

How zinc is distributed?

Human body contains 2 to 2.5gram of zinc. 70% of it is in bones. There is high concentration in skin, hair and testes. In blood it is concentrated in RBCs and platelet. Normal blood serum levels are found 75 to 125 microgram/dl.

How zinc is being absorbed?

It is absorbed in upper part of small intestine but little is known about its mechanism. It appears to be regulated in cells of intestinal walls. Absorption decreases as stores of zinc increases. Phytic acid and fiber decreases its absorption. Non-heme inorganic iron interferes its absorption if iron/zinc ratio reaches 2:1. Human milk has zinc-binding substance to enhance its absorption. Very small amount is lost in urine.

What is the biological role of zinc?

- It is a essential part of 40enzymes involved in digestion and metabolism.

- It is essential as carbonic enhydrase in RBCs.
- It maintains acid/base balance.
- It plays role in protein digestion.
- As a part of alkaline phosphatase it is involved in bone, heart, kidney and placental metabolism.
- Its most critical role is as a integral part of DNA and RNA.

How it is related to reproduction?

In rats it has been proved that its deficiency results in infertility. In humans prenatal deficiency may result in deficit learning and low birth weight. Humans may result in retarded gonadal development in males and impaired sexual maturity in both sexes.

What is the role of zinc in health of skin?

It has been associated with wound healing. Inclusion of zinc sulphate in diet avoids acne. It is also useful in treatment of dermatitis enteropathica characterized by dermatitis, diarrhoea and hair loss. Low level of zinc may result in skin rashes.

Does its deficiency affects sense of taste and smell?

Yes, loss of sense of taste is associated with loss of appetite. There is a loss of smell also.

What are other role of zinc?

- It is essential in normal glucose tolerance.
- It plays a role in mobilization of vitamin A from its storage site in liver.
- Zinc is useful in the treatment of sickle cell anemia.

What is the daily requirement of zinc?

Daily requirement is 15mg and 5mg is recommended to ensure that 0.75mg becomes available to growing fetus and placenta.

Recommended dietary allowance for zinc

Group	Zinc
Infants	3 to 5mg
Children 1 – 10 yrs	10mg
Males	15mg
Females	15mg
Pregnant	20mg
Lactating	25mg

What foods are rich source of zinc?

Dietary source of zinc mg / 100 gram

Food	Zinc	Food	Zinc
Beans	42	Cashewnut	4
Potatoes	0.9	Chicken	2.9
Peas	0.7	Whole wheat	3.9
Wheat germ	16.7	Pork	1.9
Spinach	0.2	Oils	0.8
Almonds	2.6	Cabbage	0.2

How to test zinc deficiency?

Hair analysis will tell about its deficiency. Similarly the level of zinc in saliva, skin and fingernails may give indication. Taste acquity is not a reproducible test.

COPPER

The presence of copper was first recognized in 1875. Human body contains 100 to 150mg of copper. Traces of copper are found in all tissues. Highest concentration is found in liver, brain and heart.

How is copper absorbed and metabolized?

40 to 60% ingested copper is absorbed. It is taken up rapidly from stomach and upper intestine. Absorbed copper appears in blood with in 15 minutes. It is excreted through feces and urine.

Vitamin C can cause its decreased absorption.

What are the functions of copper?

- Its role is in preventing anemia.
- It is effective in synthesis of heme.
- It is a part of multifunctional enzyme known as ceruloplasmin or feroxidase I or II.
- Several copper containing proteins erythroeuprein protects against the toxin effects of oxygen.

What is the daily requirement of it?

2 to 3mg per day is considered safe and sufficient, 1 to 3mg is suggested intake for children.

What are good food sources of it?

It depends on copper content of soil where it has been produced. Among rich sources are organ meats, Whole gram cereals, legumes, and nuts. Milk is a poor source of it.

What are the signs of copper deficiency?

Dietary deficiency is not very common. Low levels of copper have been seen in kwashiorkor and nephritic syndrome.

In excess amount copper is toxic and may deposit in liver, brain and other organs. Excess copper leads to hepatitis, renal dysfunction and lenticular degeneration resulting in Wilson's disease.

FLUORINE

Fluoride occurs in body as a calcium salt in bones and teeth. Water level of 1 part fluoride per million may reduce the incidence of dental cavities. Fluoride maintains bony structure. Fluoride salts or calcium are less easily lost preventing osteoporosis.

How is fluorine metabolized?

These are absorbed from gastrointestinal tract. Most of ingested fluoride is excreted in urine. Average daily excretion is 3mg.

What is the estimated safe intake?

Intake of 1.5 to 4.0mg per day for adults is safe. Infants should have a daily intake of 0.1 to 1.0mg.

What are its food sources?

Fluoride occurs in all soils, plants and animals. It is a normal constituent of diet. Six glasses of water containing 1 ppm will provide an additional 1.2mg.

What will happen if excess of fluoride is consumed?

Chronic dental fluorosis results when the concentration of fluoride in drinking water is in excess of 2.0ppm. Teeth will become mottled and enamel will become dull and pitting.

Excess of fluorine 20 – 80mg daily for several years will lead to bone fluorosis-resembling arthritis.

SELENIUM

It is present in all tissues. Maximum amount is found in kidney, liver, spleen, pancreas and testes. Blood level remains 25μgm per 100ml. In malnutrition children level is found below 11μgm percent.

What is the function of Selenium?

It acts as an antioxidant. Selenium is an integral part of enzymes glutathione peroxide, which deactivates lipid peroxides.

What are the rich sources of selenium?

Seafood and meat are rich sources of selenium. Cereals also contribute a lot. There becomes a little loss in milling. Vegetables and fruits are poor sources of it.

What is the daily requirement of it?

Estimated safe and adequate intake ranges from 0.05 to 0.2mg selenium per day. For infants requirement is 0.12mg.

What are the deficiency signs of it?

In humans definite deficiency signs are not known. In animals faulty development of vascular systems, cataracts and degeneration of pancreas is noted.

What are its toxic symptoms?

Stiffness, blindness, loss of hair have been noted in animals.

CHROMIUM

Adult body contains about 5mg chromium. Plasma chromium is 3 pats per billion.

What are the rich sources of chromium?

High concentration in hair, spleen, kidney and testes. Lower concentrations are available in heart, pancreas, lungs and brain.

How much chromium is absorbed?

Usable form of chromium is the glucose tolerance factor. Absorption is 10 to 25% of GFT. Only 1% of inorganic chromium is absorbed.

What are the functions of chromium?

- Glucose tolerance factor is essential for the efficient use of insulin.
- It enhances removal of glucose from blood.
- It is associated with RNA.
- It is also an activator of several enzymes.

What are its deficiency signs?

Deficiency generally develops in old age, diabetes and in infants with malnourishment.

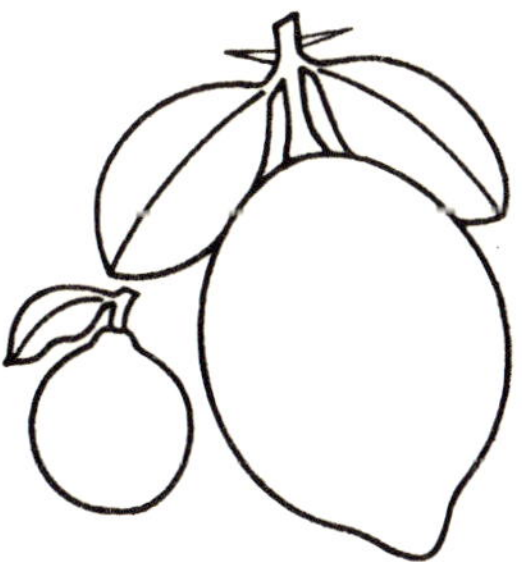

Water

Water is the main solvent in the body. Body's need for water is second to oxygen. One can live without food but without water is not feasible. 10% of loss of body water is a serious hazard and one may even die.

How is water distributed in body?

Water makes upto 50 to 70% of weight of human body. Thin people have a higher percentage of body water than fatty person. Young have a higher ratio of water than older. All tissues contain water.

What are fluid compartments?

Body fluid is in two compartments. Intracellular fluid is that which exists within the cells. It accounts for 45% of body weight. The extra cellular fluid is subdivided as follows

I. Plasma fluid accounts for 5% of body weight.

II. Interstitial fluid accounts for 15% of body weight.

What are the functions of water?

- Water is the structural component and cushion for all cells.
- Each gram of protein holds 4gm of water.
- Each gram of fat is associated with 0.2gm of water.
- It is the part of digestive juices, blood, urine and sweat.
- Water is solvent of nutrients and waste.
- Water regulates body temperature.
- Each liter of water lost in perspiration represents a heat loss of 600kcal.

- Water is essential as a body lubricant.

What are important sources of water?

Body gets water by direct ingestion orally and by oxidation of foodstuffs.

Important sources of water

Food	% water content
Milk	87
Eggs	73
Meat	40
Fruits / vegetables	70 – 90
Cereals Raw	1 – 5
Cereals cooked	80%
	Bread 35%

What is the daily loss of water?

Daily loss of water includes

Urine	1000 – 1500
Feces	100 – 200
Lungs	250 – 400
Insensible perspiration	400 – 600

What are renal losses?

Loss of water from kidney along with urine, urea and sodium chloride takes place.

How water balance is maintained?

Normal Water balance

Available	Water	Excreted	Water
Water	1200ml	In urine	1350
Water in food	900	In Stool	200
Water of oxidation	250	From Skin	400
Total	2350		2350

Balanced Diet

It is a diet which takes are of nutrients required by body + a little reserve to meet requirement in case of lean period.

Balanced diet for different sex and age group

Food Item	Adult Man			Adult Woman			Children		Boys	Girls
	Sedentary Work	Moderate Work	Heavy Work	Sedentary Work	Moderate Work	Heavy Work	1-3 yrs	4-6 yrs	10-12 yrs	10-12 yrs
Cereals	460	520	670	410	440	575	175	270	420	380
Pulses	40	50	60	40	45	50	35	35	45	45
Leafy vegetables	40	40	40	100	100	50	40	50	50	50
Others vegetables	60	70	80	40	40	100	20	30	50	50
Roots and tubers	50	60	80	50	50	60	10	20	30	30
Milk	150	200	250	100	150	200	300	250	250	250
Oil and fat	40	45	65	20	25	40	15	25	40	35
Sugar or Jaggery	30	35	55	20	20	40	30	40	45	45

Suggested substitution for non vegetarian

Food item which can be deleted from non Vegetarian diet	Substitution than can be suggested for deleted item or items
5% of pulses (20– 30 gm)	1. One egg or 30 gm of meat or fish. 2. Addition 5 gm of fat or oil.
10% of pulses (40–60 gm)	1. Two eggs or 50 gm of meat or fish or one egg+ 30 gm of meat or fish 2. 10 gm of fat or oil.

Additional allowances during pregnancy and lactation

Food Items	During Pregnancy	Calories (Keal)	During Lactation	Calories (Keal)
Cereal	35 gm	118	60 gm	203
Pulses	15 gm	52	30 gm	105
Milk	100 gm	83	100 gm	83
Fat	–	–	10 gm	90
Sugar	10	40	10 gm	40
Total		293		521

Religion and Food Practices

Religion is a belief system including the myths that explain the social and religious order and rituals. Through it community carries out their beliefs.

Can sacrificing of food be a source communicating with God?

Sacrifices to Gods are common ways to avoid undesirable events to ensure rains, For the welfare of oneself parents use to sacrifice even their younger children. Later on it gave way to animal or plants sacrifices. Generally goat used to be slaughtered. Later on people used to gather to eat slaughtered animal as 'prashad'.

Can leaving food be taken as rejecting wordliness?

Self-denial of food is highly valued or promoted in many religious codes. Observing fast is the worldwide phenomenon in one form or the other. Fasting in Hinduism is a way to free soul from wordly matters and attraction. Fasting was thought to be a way to come to near the God.

Can food practices enhance belongingness?

Food practices may demonstrate social boundaries. Hindu system permits and imposes only pure i.e. vegetarian food to Brahmins and business community. Mohammedan prohibits pork to be eaten as Hindus prohibits cow slaughtering. Once. Pope Gregory III prohibited horse flesh to Christians. Some of these rules apply to every day eating and or on specific occasions. In medieval Japan the event of Buddhism resulted in prohibition of meat eating. Deer became mountain – whale and seal whale was considered a fish, which was then banned?

What is fasting?

A fast may mean leaving only certain categories of food or it may mean denial of meal except water. Fasting may be during daytime as in Ramjan where it is compensated eating at night. In Hindus some don't consume meat on Tuesdays. Catholics subsitituents fish for meat on Fridays. Certain festivals involve not using common salts and on certain days people take only fruits.

What are the common dietary restrictions in different religions?

Food restrictions

Islam	No Blood No Pork No Liquor
Jainism	No Non Vegetarian food
Sikhism	No Beef
Hindusm	Not to kill animals for the sake of eating
Judaism	Eat only fish – scales and fins, no blood, eat only forequarters of an animals
Time of the day	
Islam	Food not to be consumed between sunrise and sunset during ramjan
Budhism	Monks do not eat after midday
Jainism	Don't eat after sunset
Days of Year	
Judasim	No food preparation on Sabbath
Christinity	No meat on Fridays during lent
Greek orthodox	Fast Wednesday and Fridays
Hinduism	No meat on Tuesdays and during navratri and shradhs.

What is the effect of Islam on food habbit?

Islam is one of the youngest of major religions. They believe that Mohammed was the last of god's prophet.

All foods are permitted with a few exceptions that are specifically prohibited. Flesh of animals that are cloven hoofed and those that chew the cud is permitted. Pigs, blood and foods offered to other ideals are forbidden, though one who eats under constraint does not commit sin. Alcohol is prohibited. Fish must be alive when taken from sea and only fish, which have fins and scales, are allowed. Land animals without ears i.e. frogs and snakes are prohibited. To be acceptable to Muslims an animal must be bleed to death while the words, Bismillah Allah Akbar, are spoken. Such type of meat is known as 'halal'

Mohammad recommended fast on Monday and Thursday of every week and on 13th, 14th and 15th day of each month. Ramjan falling in the 9th lunar month is the major fast of the year. Fasts burn away sin. Special dish are prepared to celebrate Roza Khushai, the day of Childs first fast. The days fast should be broken as soon as sunsets by a snack known as Iftari. Younger children are expected to take short fasts.

Id is associated with serving of sweet foods and is known as 'Sweet Id'. That day sawaiyan are distributed. It provides an opportunity of food sharing, equality and hospitability for guest 'Id-ul-azan' or bakra Id is celebrated two and half months later when annual pilgrimage to Macca is underway. Bakra Id features a blood sacrifice called quarbani. Liver, lungs and heart of an animal and are removed to prepare' Kaleji '

What type of food is preferred by Judaism?

Only animals having cloven hooves and that chew cud parts are permitted. Thus cows, sheep and goats may be eaten while pigs, hares and camels are not permitted. Permitted fish must have fins and scales excluding shellfish. Winged insects and certain birds are forbidden; blood and fatty organs are not permitted.

Animals dying of natural cause or of disease are not allowed. Meat must be obtained from animals, which are being slaughtered ritually. A trained butcher slashes the animals throat with a single cut allowing whole blood to come out of dead body. After slaughter soaking, draining and salting of meat ensures all tracts of blood out. Meat was prohibited to be mix with milk.

Sabbath is a day of rest, all food preparations are carried on Friday. Rosh Hashannah the Day of Judgment is the jewish New Year Festival. Sweet foods such as apple slice dipped in honey are eaten.

During the sedar meal a collection of strolls and prayers known as Haggadah is read. Foods on the sedar dish are eaten at specific points during this reading. A dish of salt water into which the parsley is dipped symbolizes the tears of the oppressed. Four cups of wine are drunk during the meal recalling the four promises of redemption given in exodus and a fifth cup is filled for the prophet Elijah, who is said to visit every Jewish home on this night.

What type of food Hinduism favours?

Dietary laws were recorded in the code of Manu in the second centuary. Over 200foods and food related activities were forbidden. Meat eating is discouraged. Dietary regulations were including –

- One should cease from eating all flesh. There is no fault in eating flesh, nor in drinking intoxicating liquor, nor in copulation, for that is the occupation of beings but cessation from that produces great fruit.

- Meat can never be obtained without injury to living creatures and injury to sentient beings is detrimental to the attainment of heavenly bliss.
- Caste systems affects food practices. It determines what and with whom one can eat. Eating with or accepting food from members of lower castes was discouraged. Wealthy families can have two kitchens one for brahamins and another for non-brahamins.
- Food has been categorized as pukka and katacha food. Katcha foods are rice and chapaties and are most vulnerable to impurity. While pukka foods are deep fried in ghee and are pollution free.
- Devout vegetarian are Hindus. Meat, fish and eggs are avoided strictly. There are hundred of festival days celebrated in different parts of India. Some are national and some are regional. Food offered to God is blessed one and is distributed to eager crowd.

Do Sikhs also observe some food restrictions?

Sikhs means disciple, a follower of ten Gurus. It was founded in 15th century by Gurunanak. Gurunanak rejected the social system of caste pattern and idol worship. Those who sought him had first to eat in a Kitchen where all caste sat side by side to eat. Guru Gobind Singh prebade tobacco and alcohol as well as meat from animals which has bled to death. They do not eat beef. Permitted animal must be killed with a single blow known Jhatka.

Does Buddhism permit to kill animals?

Buddhism developed as an offshoot from Hinduism found in sixth century. B.C by Siddharth Gautam. No solid food may be eaten in afternoon. Five pungent foods, garlic, scallion, leek, chives and onion are to be avoided as they create great emotions, which interface with the purification of mind. Fish found dead in water may be eaten. The twin concepts of karma or moral, conduct and karuna or compession underlie. Buddhist practice vegetarianism. The karmic concept that good is rewarded by good and evil with evil leads to belief a life destroyed must be payed with life and thus the path of Nirvan is delayed. Monks prefer obtaining of food through begging only.

What restrictions are being put on food by Jainism?

It is an ascetic religion whose adherent advocates ahimsa or non injury both as an ethical or philosophical goal. Monks carry a small brush with which they carefully sweep the floor before sitting or lying so as to avoid crushing of insects. A mask may be worn to prevent inhalation of small creatures. They beg for food. They are pure vegetarians.

Do Africans also believe in myths of food?

There one of the important rituals is that of animals sacrifice. Sacrifice is associated with the agricultural calender with medical curative needs and with divination rituals. Animals with particular colour and size are more or less suitable for specific deities. These are offered in return for blessings or perhaps to effect cures or avert death in one who is ill.

Different Foods

Food can by classified into cereals, green leafy vegetables, roots and tubers, milk & milk products etc.

CEREALS

What is the composition of wheat?

It is a stable diet in North India. It contains 70% starch, 8 to 12 % gluten and 15% water. The seed or Kernel of the cereal grain is divided into 3 parts, bran, germ and endosperm. The aburone layer is just below the bran. The average composition of whole grain is protein 12, fat 2, carbohydrate 75% water 10 plus minerals phosphorus and iron.

How many calories wheat provides?

Cereals are primary source of energy for most of Indians. On an average wheat provides 350 calories per 100 gm.

What is the nutritive value of wheat?

Showing composition of wheat products per 100 gram.

	Protein (gm)	Fat (gm)	Fiber (gm)	Iron (mg)	B1(mg)
Whole wheat flour	11.8	1.5	1.2	5.3	0.54
Maida	10.2	0.8	0.2	1.5	0.12
Suji	10.4	0.8	0.2	1.6	0.12

Wheat is not a good source of calcium, vitamin – C and vitamin – A.

What is white flour?

Maida consists of endosperm of wheat and is practically free from bran. It is of good taste and biscuits are made out of it. It results in constipation and is inferior to whole wheat atta.

What is suji?

It is simply a coarse grain derived from outer coat of wheat. It is rich in protein, minerals and vitamin B1. Cooking causes loss of 33% of thiamine during chapatti making. Puri frying looses 40 to 90 % of it . Wheat is poor in lysine and 10 to 30 % of it is lost during bread making.

Is rice more nutritious?

It is a staple diet of south and East Indians, Chinese and Japanese. The pericarp and embryo are rich in B-complex. It is rich in starch and hence is eaten with nitrogen and fatty substances like pulses, fish, meat etc.

What is the composition of wheat bran?

It is the outer brown layer and it contains,

- Bulk forming carbohydrates
- B- vitamins
- Minerals specially iron

What is the nutritive value of wheat germ?

Germ is the heart of wheat known as embryo too. It contains—

- Protein comparable to proteins of meat / milk
- Vitamin B1 and vitamin E
- Iron

RICE

Describe the composition of rice?

Outer layer of pericarp contains vitamin B1 and its complete removal may give rise to beriberi in rice eating community. Rice does not contain vitamin A,C & D. Hand pounding of rice removes 25 % thiamine and machine milling removes 75% of it.

What about rice carbohydrates?

Carbohydrates which give energy to body constitue about 80% of rice in form of starch. Starch is a complex carbohydrate made up of glucose units. Glucose derived from starch is the main source of energy. Starches when eaten in a cooked form are completely digested.

Can oil by derived from rice bran?

National institute of Nutrition has certified that this oil is toxicologically safe for human consumption. It is richer in vitamin E which gives oxidative stability to oil. It has higher colesterol lowering effect and keeping quality is higher- In process of deep frying, less of this oil is being absorbed.

What is parboiling of rice?

Perboiling of paddy has been used for centuries. It is steamed by a special process so that thiamin and other vitamins and minerals are distributed through out kernel. Washing and cooking also causes a slight loss.

Showing food value of different types of rice 100 gram.

Nutrients	Parboiled Rice Hand-Pounded	Milled	Raw Rice Hand-Pounded	Milled	Rice Bran	Rice Flakes	Rice Puffed
Protein (g.)	8.5	6.4	7.5	6.8	13.5	6.6	7.5
Carbohydrates(g)	77.4	79.0	76.7	78.2	48.4	77.3	73.6
Fat (g)	0.6	0.4	1.0	0.5	16.2	1.2	0.1
Energy (Kcal)	394	346	346	345	393	346	325
Vitamins							
Carotene (ug)	9	-	2	0	-	0	0
Thiamine (mg	0.27	0.21	0.21	0.06	2.70	0.21	0.21
Riboflavin (mg)	0.12	0.05	0.16	0.06	0.48	0.05	0.01
Niacin (mg)	4.0	3.8	3.9	1.9	29.8	4.0	4.1
Pyridoxine (mg)	-	0.24	-	-	-	-	-
Folic acid (ug)	-	11.0	-	8.0	-	-	-
Vitamin C (mg)	0	0	0	0	0	0	0
Minerals							
Calcium (mg)	10	9	10	10	67	20	23
Iron (mg)	2.8	1.0	3.2	0.7	35.0	20.0	6.6
Fibre (g.)	-	0.2	0.6	0.2	4.3	0.7	0.3

Rice is generally washed and then cooked in excess of water. The gruel present is drained off and lot of B1 is lost.

What is the nutritional value of maize?

It is a stable diet of poor class Indians. It contains sufficient quantity of carbohydrate but lacks in essential aminoacid tryptophan. Deficiency of tryptophan leads to pellagra. It also lacks in gluten so it does not form a smooth chapatti hence wheat atta or milk has to be added.

Composition of different food – cereals per 100/gm.

Food	Protein (gm)	Fat (gm)	Calcium (mg)	Iron (mg)	Nicotinic Acid (mg)	Calories
Bajra	11.6	5.0	50	8.8	2.3	360
Maize	11.9	3.6	50	3.8	1.2	374
Ragi	7.1	1.3	33	5.4	1.1	332
Jowar	10.4	1.9	25	5.8	2.3	330

What about Bajra?

It is consumed as a regular food item in many Asian and African countries. It contain 11.6 % protein and better minerals than rice. It is a good source of iron too.

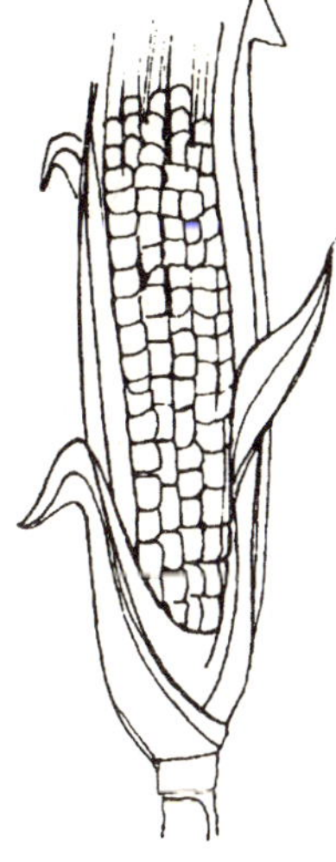

PULSES

Why pulses are known as poor man's meat?

Cost wise proteins of pulses are cheaper than proteins of animal origin per unit. These contain 20 to 25 % protein more than meat, egg and fish, although these are class- two proteins.

Pulses contain fair amount of minerals like calcium and iron. Pulses are rich in lysine and poor in sulpher containing methionine but when taken along with wheat- bread then it compensates for the deficiency of lysine of wheat and thus improves the quality of protein.

What is the composition of pulses gm / 100 gm?

Composition of pulses gm / 100 gm

Dal	Protein	Fat	Calcium gm	Iron mg	Calories value
Masoor	25.1	0.7	0.13	2.0	540
Moong	24.0	1.3	0.14	8.4	334
Chana	17.0	5.3	0.14	8.8	316
Arhar	21.3	1.7	0.14	8.8	333
Dry peas	19.7	1.1	0.07	4.4	315
Beans	24.9	0.8	0.06	2.0	337
Soya bean	40.0	20.0	0.20	6.7	432

Why soya bean has become so popular?

For a poor person soya bean is a boon at cheaper rate to get high protein, high fat and rich calories.

Protein content of soya bean is 40 % which is more than of 18 % of meat and three times that of eggs (13.3 %), four times of wheat (11 %) and other cereals. Other pulses contain 20 – 25 % of proteins. Although quality of soya – protein may be little inferior to that of milk and eggs.

What are other nutritional sources of soya bean?

From 18 to 20 % of the dry bean is an oil of sulpher quality. It contains 20 % of carbohydrate, only 11 % of this is in the form of starch and is utilized by body. For this reason it can be used by diabetics too.

Dry bean is an excellent source of thiamine, riboflavin and niacin Green beans provide vitamin 'A' and vitamin 'C' also.

What are the mineral contents of soya bean?

Soya bean contains practically all the essential minerals in adequate quantity. It has four times as much sodium and potassium as does wheat and five times as much phosphorus. Mineral ash is alkaline and becomes beneficial in balancing high acidic diet containing cereals. Wheat flour is acidic, substituting soya bean flour will help to balance the acid.

How much aminoacid soya bean contains?

Except for a deficiency of methionine and cystine soya bean is well balanced in respect of aminoacids. On heating availability of methionine as well as cystine increases and hence quality of protein improves. Soya bean is a good source of lysine. It is heat resistant.

What is the nutritive value of soya bean?

Raw soya bean possesses a low nutritive value due to presence of heat labile trypsin inhibitor and protein fraction known as soyin. Germination improves the quality of protein.

How many calories soya bean provides?

As regards calories one pound of whole soya bean flour is equivalent to three quartz of milk or twenty nine eggs, or three and a half pound of beef steak. As regards to protein one pound of soya bean is equivalent to two pounds of beef steak, two and half dozen eggs or six quarters of milk.

What is the supplementary value of soya bean?

Being rich in both lysine and valine it is efficient in supplementing wheat protein which lacks in lysine.Bread containing soya bean is superior in the quality of proteins of wheat bread. Optimally heat processed soya bean is superior to Bengal gram in its supplementary value.

Can soya – milk be used?

Yes, soya milk can be made

- 2 litres of water
- 1 cup soya bean flour
- 1 tea spoon ful suger
- ¼ tea spoonful salt.

Mix the flour first with a little of water to make a smooth paste.Add rest of water slowly in 5 minutes. Stir and watch to avoid burning of fire. Strain through a fine cloth. This milk will keep as long as animal milk.

Composition of different milk per 100 / gm

Nutrient	Soya been milk	Groundnut Milk	Cow's Milk
Protein (gm)	2.4	3.0	3.2
Fat (gm)	2.5	5.2	4.9
Carbohydrate (gm)	3.2	3.1	4.6
Calcium (gm)	0.08	0.11	0.11
Iron (mg)	1.2	1.4	0.2
Caloric value	51	71	75

If you need milk rich in fat and protein more of soya flour can be used.

ROOTS/TUBERS

What about vegetables

These are reserve of nutrients for use of plant itself. They are poor source of proteins and fats hence are inferior to cereals. They contain salts of potash.

Composition of roots / tubers per 100 gram

	Protein gm	Fibre gm	Iron mg	Vit C mg	Calcium mg	Calories
Carrot	0.9	1.2	2.2	3	30	47
Potato	1.9	0.4	0.7	17	10	97
Turnip	0.5	0.9	0.4	43	30	29
Radish	0.7	0.8	0.4	15	50	17
Onion	1.8	0.6	1.2	2	40	59
Colocasia	3.0	1.0	1.7	-	40	97
Beatroot	1.7	0.9	0.4	43	200	43

FRUITS

What is the importance of fruits?

These are used either as food or as a flavering agent.

As food they contain mineral salts and easily assimiable form of carbohydrate such as levulose and fructose. Salts of potash combined with vegetable acid help in maintaining alkaline reserve of body. Unripe fruits may irritate bowels but as fruit ripens starch is converted into sugar and acid.

Flavour of fruits depends on content of volatile oil.

Are costly fruits the best nutritionally?

Costly fruits are not necessarily the best one. Banana is the cheapest when considered as a food than fruit. Grapes and apples are not of high nutrition value. Various fruit guices are palatable drinks.

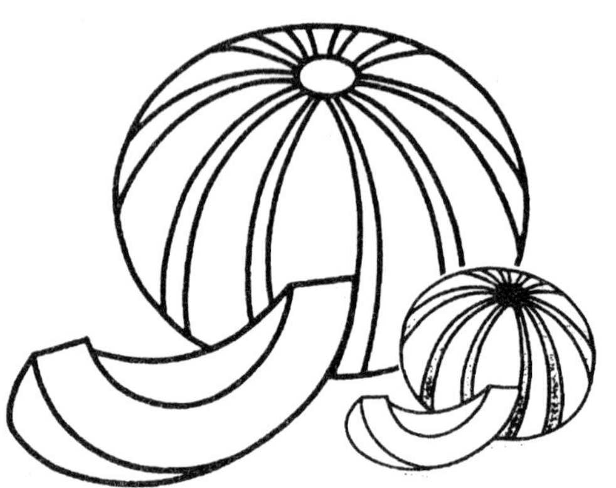

Is banana a healthier food?

It is a poor man's food. Ripe fruit is a rich source of carbohydrates, minerals and B complex. Composition varies with type and stage of maturity. Every part of banana tree, fruit and flower is edible. Ripening takes place usually 30 – 48 hours in a cool store. Ripening takes place well at about 15 degree 'C' to 20 degree 'C'. The application of Vaseline or coaltar to the cut ends of stalks prevents rottening. Ethylene gas may be used for early repening.

Starch constitutes the major carbohydrate of green banana. As fruit repens, starch is rapidly hydrolyzed into soluble sugers and percentage of total suger increases 1 – 2 in green banana to 15 – 20 in ripe fruit. It contains 350 volatile oils giving flavours. Banana contains large amount of serotinin and norepinephrine. Serotinin inhibits gastic secretion and stimulates smooth muscles. Norepinephrine is vasoconstricting agent. Banana is useful in constipation and peptic ulcer.

Nutritive value of banana (ripe), plantain (green), plantain flower, plantain stem (per 100 gms of edible portion)

	Banana	Plantain Flower	Plantain (green)	Plantain (Stem)
Moisture (g)	70.1	89.9	83.2	88.3
Protein (g)	1.2	1.7	1.4	0.5
Fat (g)	0.3	0.7	0.5	0.1
Fibre (g)	0.4	1.3	0.7	0.8
Carbohydrates (g)	27.2	5.1	14.0	9.7
Energy (Kcal)	116.0	34.0	64.0	42.0
Calcium (mg)	17.0	32.0	10.0	10.0
Phosphorous (mg)	36.0	42.0	29.0	10.0
Iron (mg)	0.36	1.6	6.3	1.1
Vitamins				
Carotene (mg)	78.0	27.0	30.0	0
Thiamine (mg)	0.05	0.05	0.05	0.02
Riboflavin (mg)	0.04	0.02	0.02	0.01
Niacin (mg)	0.6	0.4	0.3	0.2
Vitamin C (mg)	32.0	16.0	24.0	7.0
Minerals(mg/100g)				
Magnesium	41.0	54.0	13.0	-
Sodium	36.6	20.1	15.0	-
Potassium	88.0	185.0	193.0	-
Zinc	0.15	-	0.05	-

What is the composition of fruits?

Composition of fruits per 100 gram

	Protein gm	Fat gm	Carbohydrate gm	Vit. A I, Unit	Vit C mg	Calories
Apple	0.3	0.1	13.4	Trace	2	56
Banana	1.2	0.3	36.4	Trace	1	116
Grape	0.1	0.2	10.2	15	31	45
Mango	0.6	0.1	11.8	800	13	50
Papaya	0.5	0.1	9.5	2020	46	40
Jack fruit	1.9	0.1	19.9	540	10	84
Lemon	1.0	0.9	11.1	Trace	33	57

ANIMAL FOODS

Meat consists of muscle fibers held together by connective tissue. Proteins of meat are myosin, muscle albumin and myoglobin. These proteins are class one proteins which are easily digested.

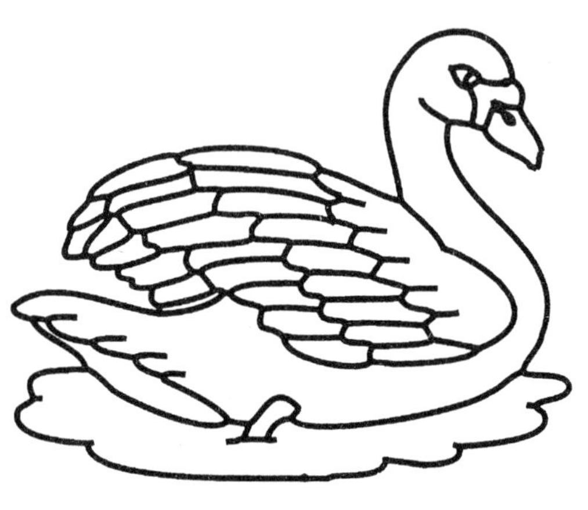

When meat should be consumed?

Rigor mortis (rigidness) develops in meat due to clotting of myosin but acids which develop soon soften the myosin and make the meat tender and give it a bitter flavour. Hence meat should be eaten after rigor mortis has set in and passed away.

On boiling the collagen of the meat is gelatinized. The connective tissue is much more abundant in aged animals so it becomes more tough and takes more time for cooking. Hence meat of younger animal is preferred being softer.

What are the qualities of good meat?

- It should be firm and elastic to touch
- It should have little or no odour
- It should not shrink or waste much on cooking. It should not leave water
- It should have marble appearance due to remification of veins amongst muscles
- Pale pink colour is a sign of disease

When meat start to putrefy it becomes pale, moist, doughy, smells sickly and offensive and gradually turns greenish. It becomes soft and is torn easily on stretching.

What is the composition of different types of meat?

Composition of animal food gm / 100gm

Food	Protein gm	Fat gm	Vit A I. Units	Calcium mg	Calories
Beef	22.6	2.6	59	10	114
Mutton	18.5	13.3	31	150	194
Fish	19.2	3.9	-	530	112
Pork	18.7	4.4	-	30	114
Egg	13.3	13.3	1200	60	173

What type of meat is easily digestible?

Cooking sterilizes the meat and kills parasites. Meat being a bad conductor should be cooked slowly and for prolonged period. Mutton is more easy to digest because its fibers are shorter and more tender but contains more fat.

The fibers of goat flesh are shorter, more tender than beef and contains less fat. Hence goat flesh is more easily digested. The flesh of partrige is white, tender having delicate fiber and flavour and easy to digest. Flesh of ducks and geese is darker and is well known to disagree with delicate stomach. Game birds contain less fat and largely eaten as delicate food.

Liver of an animal is rich in vitamin A, B, C, and D, especially vitamin A. Liver protein is digested comfortably and contains manganese and iron.

How meat can be preserved?

There can be many methods to preserve the meat, such as

(1) Heat – It is used in the process of canning. During it vitamin 'C' is destroyed.

(2) **Refrigeration** – Cold prevents the growth and multiplication of bacteria.

(3) **Salting and pickling** – Meat is smeared with salt. It does superficial preservation for a short period while pickling.

(4) **Smoking**- Meat is salted and then hang up in a big hall and exposed to smoke. Creosite present in wood-smoke kills bacteria and even spores.

What diseases can be spread by meat?

Following diseases can be spread by unhealthy meat

- **Liver flukes** – Each is 2-4 cms long and 1 cm wide, brownish in colour and found in sheeps. Parasites are found in liver.
- **Cysticercus** – Tapeworms live in the muscles of oxen and pigs where they produce cysts. In these tiny cysts lies the head of tapeworm. These head fix to intestinal wall and grow into a full grown tapeworm.

MILK AND MILK PRODUCTS

Milk is a complete and ideal food and contains most of the proximate principles in a well balanced diet.

What is the nutritive value of milk?

- It contains 3.5 % of total weight consisting of 3 % caseinogen, 0.4 % lacto albumen and 0.1 % globulin.
- Carbohydrate is the form of lactose or milk sugar. It is easily fermented by lactic acid bacilli. Human milk contains more sugar than cow milk.
- It is a poor source of vitamin C and does not contain vitamin E .
- It is a good source of calcium but is a poor source of iron.

What about milk fat?

Cow's milk contains half the fat content of buffalo milk. Fat is in the form of glycerides in emulsified form. When milk is allowed to stand for some time fat rises to the surface as cream.

Caesinogen predominates in animal milk while lactoalbumin predominates in human milk.

Does boiling preserves milk?

Boiling is a simple method adopted even at home level. By boiling organisms which produce lactic acid are being killed.

What changes are being brought by boiling?

Boiling brings the following changes in milk

- Lactoalbumin and lactoglobulin are coagulated at 160^0 F to 168^0 F respectively.
- Fat emulsion is destroyed and globules coalesce together.
- Calcium, phosphorus and magnesium are precipitated and a portion of citrate is lost.
- Vitamin 'C' is lost.
- Certain enzymes and micro organisms are destroyed.

How milk can be sterilized?

This is done by raising the temperature to 100 degree-C. and then maintaining it for 15 minutes in closed vessels. It kills all micro organisms and spores.

What do you understand by pasteurism of milk?

This process delays the natural souring of milk by 12 to 24 hours. It destroys some specific organisms such as causing tuberculosis, typhoid, cholera and dysentery.

There are many methods of pasteurization such as Holder process and Ultra High Temperature Method.

- Holder Process- Heating milk up to 150 degree 'F' and maintaining it at that temperature for 30 minutes and suddenly cooling to 55 degree 'F'.
- Ultra High Temperature Method- Milk is rapidly heated under pressure to 125 degree 'C' to 150 degree 'C' for a few seconds only and then is rapidly cooled down.

What is the advantage of Pasteurization?

- It kills 90 % bacteria
- It preserves taste, flavour, appearance and digestibility.
- Level of pasteurization is judged by phosphatase test.

How milk is dried in powder form?

Milk is passed over heated rollers where it is evaporated and thin film is formed which is powdered finally. This powder is easily digested by infants as the curd formed in their stomach will be more flocculent and finally devided than that of fresh milk.

What is condensed milk?

Milk is usually pasteurized and is gradually heated under pressure in vaccum pans, till its watery portion is evaporated and it is reduced to a quarter of its original water.

How milk is digested?

Milk is curdled by acid of gastric juice. Digestion is helped by enzyme which makes the coagula of human milk softer and flocculated. Milk should be taken in sips to prevent formation of hard clot. Digestion of milk is completed in intestine by pancreatic juice.

How to judge pure milk?

Milk should be white with no deposit or disagreeable smell or taste. Acidity above 0.4% is appreciable in taste and curdling occurs at 0.6% acidity.

Average specific gravity of milk is 1032. Lactometer is used to determine the specific gravity but it proves to be fallacious as addition of water lowers the specific gravity and extraction of fat increases the specific gravity. So people after taking out cream add water to it.

What diseases can be conveyed by milk?

Common diseases caused by milk are

- Tubercle bacillus – It spreads from cow suffering with tuberculosis or if tuberculous cook has coughed over milk.
- Typhoid – From the hands of typhoid carrier or from typhoid infected stools through flies can infect. There are chances of infection from contaminated water used in adultering milk.
- Dysentery / Cholera – If milk man is suffering from it, costomers may also suffer from it.

Consumption of raw milk is not advised.

What are the ways of adulteration of milk?

Adulteration has become a rule instead of exception. Common methods adopted are

- Extraction of cream from milk partially or completely with or without addition of water.
- Commonest way to increase the bulk is by addition of water. If water is dirty, may spread diseases.
- Addition of skimmed milk powder with water.
- Addition of gelatin, starch or maida or arrowroot after extraction of fat to make it thick.

Is curd different than milk?

Making of curd from milk is a good example of fermentation. It is being done by micro-organisms. These multiply with great rapidity. In making curd lactose is converted into lactic acid which is sour.

What is the composition of various forms of milk?

Nutrient composition of milk and milk products (100 g edible portion)

Milk	Protein (gm)	Fat (gm)	Carbohy-drates (gm)	Energy KCal	Calcium (mg)	Phosph-orus (mg)	Iron (mg)
Ass	2.1	1.5	6.5	48	80	-	-
Buffalo	4.3	6.5	5.0	117	210	130	0.2
Cow	3.2	4.1	4.4	67	120	90	0.2
Goat	3.3	4.5	4.6	72	170	120	0.3
Human	1.1	3.4	7.4	65	28	11	-
Milk Products							
Curd (cow's milk)	3.1	4.0	3.0	60	149	93	0.2
Butter milk	0.8	1.1	0.5	15	30	30	0.1
Channa Cow's milk	18.3	20.8	1.2	265	208	138	-
Cheese	24.1	25.1	6.3	348	790	520	2.1
Khoa (whole buffalo's milk)	14.6	31.2	20.5	421	650	420	5.8
Khoa (whole Cow's milk)	20.0	25.9	24.9	413	956	613	-
Skimmed milk powder (cow's milk)	38.0	0.1	51.0	357	1370	1000	1.4
Whole milk Powder (cow's milk)	25.8	26.7	38.0	496	950	730	0.6
Butter	81.0	-	729	-	-	-	-
Ghee (cow)	100.0	-	900	-	-	-	-
Ghee (buffalo)	100.0	-	900	-	-	-	-

Source: nutritive value of Indian food, NIN, 1994

EGG

Why egg is an important source of nutrition?

Egg proteins are best in quality and are taken as standard for comparing the quality of other food proteins. Egg proteins are better absorbed and utilized by body than proteins of milk.

Hen's egg weighs about 55 to 60 gm and consist of 10.5% outer layer, 60 % white and 30 % yellow yolk. Outer shell consists of carbonate of lime, white portion is of proteins i.e. albumin and yellow yolk contains mainly fat. In addition it contains lecithin, vitamins, phosphorus, lime and iron. Iron of yolk is easily digested.

How eggs provide nutritions to body?

Two eggs can provide one fourth of the daily need of protein, one third of fat, all of vitamin B12, about 3/4th of folic acid, majority of vitamin 'A' and 20 % of other vitamins.

What about digestibility of an egg?

Digestibility of an egg depends upon the form in which it is eaten.

Light boiled ——————1 hours 45 minutes

Raw egg ———————Two hours 15 minutes

Egg full boiled and omelette——————Three hours

What is the nutrition value of an egg?

The nutrition per 100 gms of edible portion

Moisture (gm %)	72.3
Protein (gm %)	13.3
Fat (gm %)	13.3
Minerals (gm %)	1.0
Energy	173
Calcium (mg)	60
Phosphorus (mg)	220
Iron (mg)	2.1
Vitamin 'A' (microgram)	360
Thiamine (mg)	0.1
Riboflavin (mg)	0.4
Niacin (mg)	0.1
Folic acid (microgram)	78.3

What about storage of an egg?

Egg is a perishable commodity and liable for deterioration. Since shell of egg is porous it is susceptible to salmonella and other bacterial infections. At higher temperature rate of carbon dioxide loss is increased and egg appears stale within a few days. Refrigeration is the only means by which egg can be stored for long periods of time.

How to check the freshness of eggs?

To check the freshness of an egg dip in a bowl of water. If it sinks and lies on the side it is fresh. If it stands it is in a stage of deterioration. If it floats to the top, it is stale and should not be eaten.

What is the effect of cooking on egg?

Cooking not only destroys bacteria but also improves certain nutrients. For example avidin present in egg prevents absorption of biotin but cooking makes biotin available.

What about fertilized Vs unfertilized eggs?

Most of eggs produced in poultry forms and sold in market are unfertilized eggs It may be one the reason why some vegetarians are turning eggtarians.

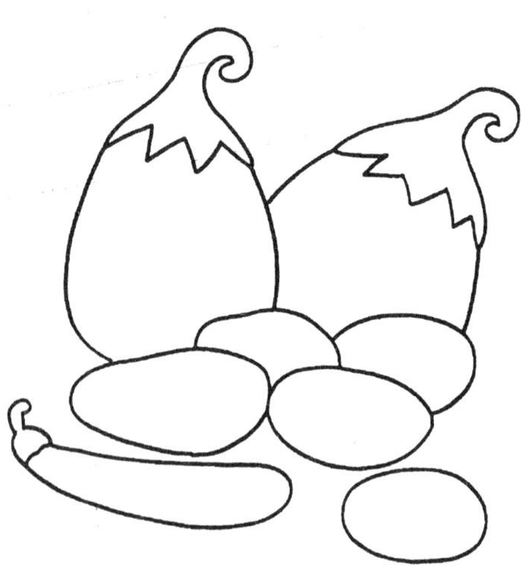

There is no difference in nutritional quality between fertilized and unfertilized eggs. Similarly colour of an egg has no bearing on nutritional quality.

Under what circumstances eggs are more helpful?

In view of high biological value and nutritive value, egg is commonly used in formulating therapeutic diets in coelic deseases. When gluten free diet has to be given eggs make a good substitute. In chronic renal failure, egg is an excellent source of protein. Eggs are useful for gastric patients since they are less acid producing than meat, fish and chicken.

What about egg cholesterol?

In recent years egg has come under some cloud because of its adverse effects in person having heart disease due to its high cholesterol level. But cholesterol is normal and essential constituent of body. It is found in blood and nervous tissue. Cholesterol is required for synthesis and proper functioning of male and female sex hormones. So cholesterol becomes very important for metabolism, body growth and development.

One cup of icecream________	50 mg of cholesterol
One egg ________________	250mg "
One cup milk ____________	35mg "
Mutton curry one Katori ____	100mg "

Liver, brain and kidney contains two to three folds of cholesterol than egg .One can consume 300 mg of cholesterol every day. One can consume 2-3 eggs per week safely if he is not consuming lot of saturated fats otherwise.

NUTS

Almond, pistachio are costlier and get place in festive diets only or in sweets.

Are nuts helpful for heart?

Nuts contain protein that is rich in arginine. It is a dietary precursor of nitric oxide, a potent endogenous vasodilator which acts as nitroglycerine. It inhibits platelet aggregation and monocyte adherence. Folic acid of nuts may help to liver homocysteine levels which is responsible for risk of coronary heart disease.

What is the nutritive values of nuts?.

Proximate principles present in 100 gms of nuts

Nuts	Calories (Kcal)	Protein (g)	Fat (g)	Fiber (g)	Calcium (g)	Iron (mg)
Almond	655	20.8	58.9	1.7	230	5.1
Cashe-wnut	596	21.2	46.9	1.3	50	4.8
Coconut (fresh)	444	4.5	41.6	3.6	10	1.7
Coconut (dry)	662	6.8	6.3	6.6	400	7.8
Gingelly seeds	563	18.3	43.3	25.0	1450	9.3
Ground nut	567	25.3	40.1	3.1	90	2.5
Pistachio nut	626	19.8	53.5	2.1	140	7.7
Walnut	687	15.6	64.5	2.6	100	2.6
Apricot (dry)	306	1.6	0.7	2.1	110	4.6
Rajgeera seeds	364	16.5	5.3	2.7	223	17.6
Makhana	347	9.7	0.1	-	20	1.4

Micronutrients present in 100 gms of nuts

Nuts	Caro tene (µg)	Thia-min (mg)	Ribofl-avin (mg)	Niacin (mg)	Folic Acid	Magne-sium	Cooper (mg)	Zinc (mg)
Almond	0	0.24	0.57	4.4	–	373	0.97	3.57
Cashewnut	60	0.63	0.19	1.2	–	349	1.66	5.99

Is coconut nutritious?

Coconut is an important food in all coconút growing countries. It is eaten raw or in puddings, sweets, curries and chutneys. A beneficial effect of adding the coconut kernel to the diet is to lower blood cholesterol.

What is the nutritive value of coconut kernel?

Nutritive Value of Kernel (per 100g)

	gm.		
Protein	3.0 - 4.5	Fiber	3.0 - 3.6
Fat	32.0 – 41.6	Mineral	0.5 - 1.0
Carbohydrate	10.0 - 15.5	Water	36.0 - 54.0
Vitamins	mg		
Vitamin E	0.2 – 0.73	Niacin	0.54
Vitamin C	1.0 -3.30	Pantothenic acid	0.30
Thiamin	0.07	Vitamin B6	0.05
Riboflavin	0.02	Folate	26.0 ug
Minerals	mg		
Calcium	14.0	Sodium	20.0
Phosphorus	113.0	Zinc	1.1
Iron	2.4	Copper	0.43
Magnesium	32.0	Manganese	1.50
Potassium	356.0	Selenium	10.1 ug
Fats (lipids)			
Total saturated fatty acids	29.7 g		
Total monounsaturated fatty acids	1.43g		
Total polyunsaturated fatty acids	0.37 g		

Can coconut milk be used?

Coconut milk is made by processing equal amounts of scraped coconut meat and water to a paste and straining out the milky liquid.

Nutritive Value Of Coconut milk (per 100 ml)

	g		
Fat	20.0 - 30.0	Minerals	0.5 - 1.0
Protein	2.5 - 3.5	Water	70.0 - 80.0
Carbohydrate	4.0 - 5.0		
Vitamins	**mg**		
Vitamin E	0.73	Pantothenic acid	0.18
Vitamin C	2.80	Vitamin B6	0.03
Thiamin	0.03	Folate	16.0 µg
Niacin		0.76	
Minerals	**mg**		
Calcium	16.0	Sodium	15.0
Iron	1.64	Zinc	0.67
Magnesium	37.0	Copper	0.27
Phosphorus	100.0	Manganese	0.92
Potassium	263.0	Selenium	6.2 µg

Coconut milk provides exotic flavour to curries and pasta dishes. It can replace cow's milk and cream in most of recipes.

What about ground nuts?

Ground nut is a concentrated source of calories like almonds and cashewnut. It is known as poor man's dry fruit. Raw ground nut contains 20 % protein and 40 % fat. Some time when ground nut is stored in humid dark place then a fungus giving rise aflatoxin which is harmful to body.

What are other nutrients available in ground nut?

Ground nuts contains no vitamin 'C' but thiamine and nicotinic acid are present in high amount. Loss may occur if seeds are roasted too much.

On the other hand protein value of ground nut in raw state is adversely affected due to heat labile trypsin inhibitor. Combination of 3/4 ground nut proteins + 1/4 milk protein becomes equivalent to class 1 proteins. High content of oil gives rise to a headache on consumption of groundnut at a stretch.

Is ground nut milk possible?

For preparing ground nut milk, seeds are soaked overnight in water and soaked seeds are ground to a paste.Six volumes of water are mixed and stirred well. After slight heating it is filtered well and boiled. Except calcium content ground nut milk is as good as ordinary milk. Curd can be made out of it.

GREEN LEAFY VEGETABLES AND GREEN TOPS

Green leafy vegetables include spinach, mustard, frence greek leaves i.e. maethee, bathua, cabbage, corianders etc. These should always be included regularly in diet. These are alkaline, rich in vitamin

'A' and 'C' and minerals like iron and calcium. Although low in calories they form roughage in our diet and are best for obese.

What about nutritive value of green leafy vegetables?

In general darker the colour of the leaves more the amount of minerals and vitamins are present. Green leaves contain chlorophyll. Whenever there is chlorophyll there is vitamin A. These contain low amount of phosphorus hence are excellent addition to our cereal diet which is high in phosphorus and low in calcium.

Nutritive value of green leafy vegetables per 100 gm

	Palak	Cholai	Sag	Maithee	Bathua	Dhania	Daily need
Vit.A (μgm)	5600	5500	1300	2300	1740	6918	750
Vit.B (μgm)	800	1500	900	1150	750	840	25
Vit C	30	100	60	50	35	135	50
Iron (mgm)	10	25	12	17	42	18	20
Calcium (μgm)	70	390	370	400	150	184	400

Can tops of certain green vegetables be used?

From following table it will be clear that green tops are more nutritious.

Showing comparative nutritive values per 100 gm. of green leaves

	Carrot leaves	Carrot	Radish leaves	Radish	Turnip leaves	Turnip	Caloca-cia leaves	Caloca-cia
Calories	77	48	38	17	67	28	56	97
Protein (gm)	5.1	9.9	3.9	0.7	4.0	0.5	3.9	3.0
Fat gm	0.5	0.2	0.6	0.1	1.5	0.2	1.5	0.1
Calcium mg	340	80	340	35	710	30	227	40
Iron mg	8.8	2.2	18	0.4	28.4	0.4	10.0	1.7
Vit A (ugm)	5700	1890	5742	3	9334	0	10270	-
Vit. C mg	79	3	106	15	180	43	112	17

How to select good leafy vegetables?

Select clean, leafy vegetables which are tender, crisp, bright green coloured, free from insects, mud spots or holes in leaves.

In head vegetables such as cabbage, the hard heavy and compact heads free from bruises and worm injuries are a good buy.

What precautions should be taken while cooking green leafy vegetables?

- If possible green fresh leaves should be used as soon as procured.

- These should be washed properly before storing or cutting.
- Thorough washing is required to remove poisonous insecticide, sprays and eggs of intestinal worms.
- Don't soak cut leaves for a long time; by doing so water soluble vitamin 'B' and 'C' will be dissolved in water and wasted.

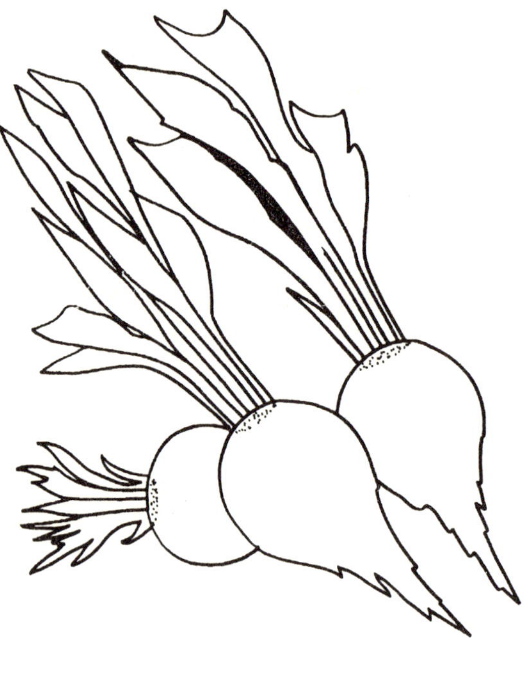

- Addition of baking powder will not only destroy the flavour but there will be a loss of vitamin B also.
- Don't cook in excess water. Avoid over cooking. Reheating creates loss of vitamin C every time.
- Boil water and then put vegetables instead of adding them to cold water and then bringing to boil.

- Adding of acidic substances like tamarind, lemon juice will reduce destruction of vitamin 'C'.

Pressure cooking is quicker and leads to conserving of nutrients being closed cooking.

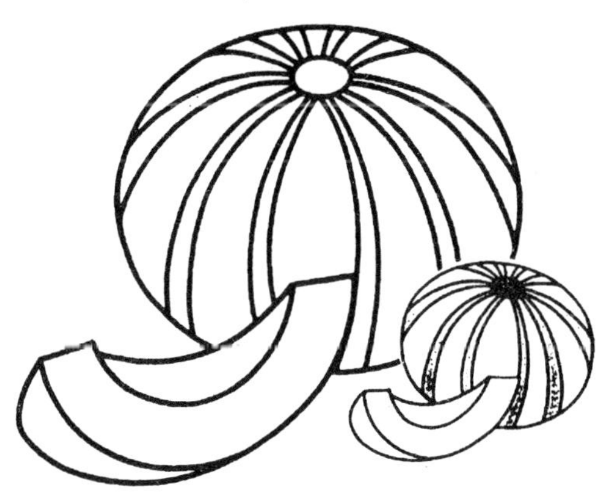

Important Food Items

BUTTER

It is prepared from milk fat by souring the cream either naturally or with bacteria followed by the churning. It contains not less than 80% fat. Rest is water. Sometime salt is being added. It contains in 100gm.

Trace of proteins

- Vitamin A – 1000μgm / 100gm.
- Vitamin D – 0.6 – 1.0μg
- Vitamin E – 2μgm

BUTTER MILK

It is a residue left after churning the butter. It contains 1 – 2% fat with other milk constituents proportionately increased. It has a acid flavour due to diacelyl.

BETEL LEAVES (PAAN)

Leaf of creeper piper betel which is chewed after food in India, Pakistan and other countries for its stimulating effect due to presence of alkaloids arecoline and guvacoline. Leaves are chewed with nuts of areca palm. It is a good source of calcium and iron.

BITTER GUARD

It is high in vitamin C, potassium, copper and iron. Its affect is alkaline. It contains a substance, which reduces blood sugar level. Fresh juices of it or of leaves or cooked vegetables all are effective.

BROCAOLI

It is high in chlorophyll and is high in protein, Vitamin C and calcium. It has no fat. Its soluble fiber with potassium and low sodium help blood pressure patient.

CAFFEINE

It is an alkaloid drug found in coffee and tea. It raises BP, stimulates kidneys and avert fatigue. Per cup of coffee contains about 100mg, Tea contains 1.5 to 2.5% caffeine and cola drink contains 3 to 4.5mg / 30ml.

CHEESE

It is prepared from cured and precipated from milk by rennin or lactic acid. Cheese is cured by being left to mature with salt under various conditions. That produces characteristic flavour of particular type of cheese.

Contents of it per 100gm are

Protein	25gm	VtaminA	20ugm
Fat	31gm	Nicotinic acid	0.1mg
Calcium	700mg		

Legally it should contain 40% fat on a dry weight.

CHOCOLATE DRINKING

It is a partly solublised cocoa for preparation of beverage including 75% sucrose.

Contents of it per 100gm are

Sugar	74gm	Fat	6gm
Starch	3.6gm	Iron	2mg
Nitrogen	1gm	Chalories	370

CLOVES

Dried flower buds of caryophyllus aromaticus. It contains 10% fix oils and a volatile oil mostly eugenol with small amounts of caryophyllene, vanillin. It is used as flavour and condiments.

Contents of it per 100gm are

Fat	22gm	Iron	10mg
Nitrogen	3.7gm	K	1500mg
Starch	12gm	Sodium	950
Calcium	130mg	Kcal	310

COCONUT

Tropical palm. Dried nut is khopra which contains 60 to 65% coconut oil. Hollow unripe nut contains are watery liquid known as coconut milk which is gradually absorbed as nut ripens.

Coconut milk contains

Solid	1.4%
Protein	0.2%
Sucrose	3%

Contents of mature kernel per 100gm

Solids	48 – 80gm	Carbohydrate	11gm
Proteins	4gm	Calories	375
Fat	35gm		

COD-LIVER OIL

Oil from codfish liver, a classical source of vitamin A&D. It contains 120 – 1200μgm vitmain A and 1 – 10μg vitaminD per gram.

CORIANDER

Dried ripe fruit of coriandrum sativum. It contains 20% fixed oil and 1% essential oil largely linool or coriandrol, used as a flavour in vegetables and meat.

CORNFLAKES

It is a breakfast cereal made out of maize.

Contents per 100gm are

Water	3gm	Protein	8gm
Sugar	7gm	Fat	0.5gm
Starch	74gm	Calorie	370
Dietary Fibre	3gm		

CORN FLOUR

It is a fatty part of milk. Light cream contains 20 – 25% fat and heavy cream 40% fat.

The cream layer forms about 6% of total depth of milk. Clotted cream contains 29.5% water, 48% fat, 4% protein, 2.8% lactose and 0.67% ash.

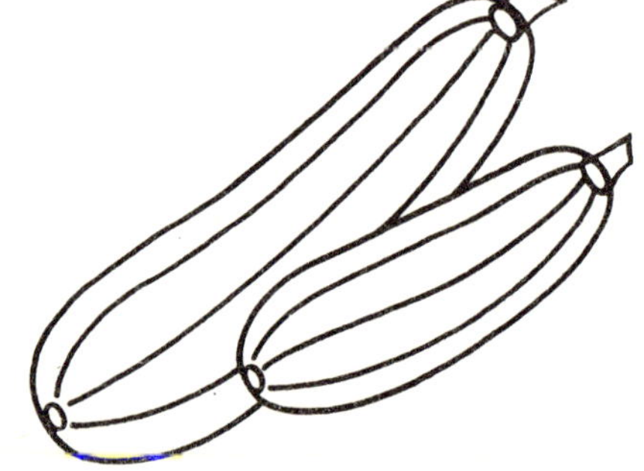

CUCUMBER

Fruit cucumis sativus.

Contents per 100gm are

Protein	0.6gm	Iron	0.2mg
Fat	0.1gm	Vitamin C	6mg
Calcium	7mg	Kcal	10

It is used as a salad and does not contain much of calories.

DATES

Fruit of date palm known as back as 3000BC. These are soft, semi dry and dry.

Contents of dry dates per 100gm are

Water	15 gm	Sugar	65gm
Dietary Fibre	9gm	Iron	1.5gm
Protein	2gm	Calories	250

EGG

It contains references proteins

Contents of egg / 100gm are

	Whole Egg	Yolk	White of yolk
Protein	12gm	16	9
Fat	11gm	31	Traces
Kcal	150	340	36
Calcium Mg	50	130	5
Iron Mg	2	0.4	Traces
Rational Mg	0.1	400µg	
Vitamin D	2µg	5µg	
Vitamin E	1.6mg	5mg	

FRENUGREEK (MAITHEE)

Leguminous plant. It is eaten as vegetable, seeds are used as a flavouring agent.

Contents 100gm

Proteins	29	Calcium	180mg
Fat	5	Iron	22mg
Carbohydrate	50	Calories	355

FIG

It is a ficous carica. It is eaten fresh / dried. It has mild luxative property.

Content of dried fig per 100gm

Protein	4gm	Iron	4mg
Carbohydrate	63gm	Vitamin A	30μgn
Calcium	200mg	Calories	270

It does not contain Vitamin C.

FISH PROTEIN CONCENTRATE

Deodorised, defatted fish meal which has been decolourised. It is a cheap sources of protein for enrichment of food. It contains 75% proteins with biological value of 75 – 80.

FRUCTOSE SYRUPS

These are glucose syrups containing more than 10% fructose. Fructose syrup may contain 35% glucose, 45% fructose and 5 – 10% maltose. They are sweet as sucrose with great viscocity. It is used in soft drinks, canned fruits and jams.

GARLIC

It is a bulb of allium sativum with pungent odour. Diallyl disulphide is responsible for characteristics odour. It lowers down cholesterol level.

GINGER

Rhizome of zingiber officinal is used as a flavour pungency due to known volatile compounds including gingerol. Ginger is preserved made from young fleshy rhizomes boiled with sugar and packed in syrup.

Contents per 100gm are

Protein	2.5gm	Fibre	2.1gm
Fat	0.8gm	Iron	2.5mg
Carbohydrate	11gm	Calories	63

GUAVA

It is a fruit of psidium guajava. It is eaten raw or preserved as a guava jelly .

Contents per 100 gm. Are

Water	80gm	Iron	1gm
Protein	1gm	Carotene	60gm
Fat	0.4gm	Vitamin C	200gm
Carbohydrate	13gm	Calories	58gm

HYDROGENATED OILS

Liquid oils can be hardened by hydrogenation. Treatment with hydrogen in the presence of nickel catalyst causes saturation raising the melting point. Sunflower and maize oils are commonly hardened.

ICE CREAMS

It is a frozen confection made from fat, milk, solid and sugars. 10% milk fat and 20% other milk solids are there. Stabilisers such as carboxy methyl cellulose, gums and alginates are included. Mono and diglycerides bind the loose globules of water. An additional and essential component of ice cream is an air. Tiny air bubbles constitute the foam. Different flavours with or without nuts are available.

JAM

Fruit preserve is set to a gel by reaction between acid, pectin and added sugar. The solution of actin in fruit is caused to conglomerate by the sugar and forms a network of fibers enclosing liquid at ph 2.5 to 3.5. Optimum sugar concentration is 67.5%. Normally 0.5 to1% pectin is used.

JELLY

A colloidal suspension that has set. It may be made from gelatin, pectin, agar and usually flavour with fruit juice.

KETCH UP

Spicy sauce or condiment made with juice of fruit or vegetables, vinegar and spices. Tomato ketch up is a common sauce.

LETTUCE

Leaves of plants lactuca sativa. Not a very valued food but is used as a salad.

Contents per 100gm are

Protein	0.9gm	Iron	0.5mg
Fat	0.1gm	Vitamin C	50mg
Carbohydrate	16gm	Calories	70

MANGO

Deep yellow colour is an index of vitamin A, which can be up to700mg per 100gm. Thousands of varieties are available.

Contents per100gm are

Protein	0.9gm	Carotene	200mg
Fat	0.5gm	Vitamin C	30mg
Carbohydrate	16gm	Calories	63
Iron	0.5mg		

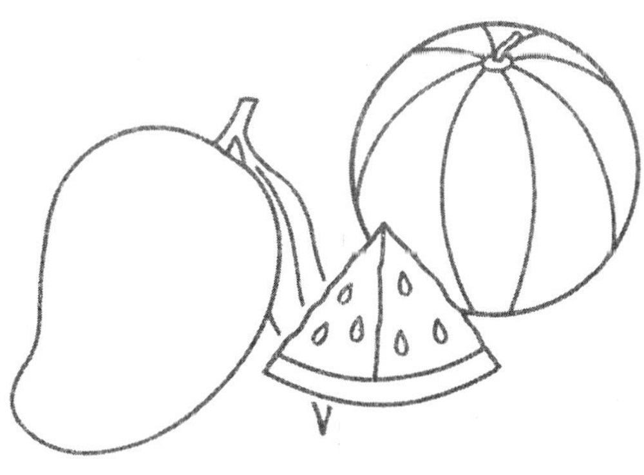

MARGRAINE

Emulsion of fat from any vegetable animal or marine oils with 16% water, flavoured and colourful. Soft margrines are usually rich in polyunsaturated fatty acid. It is generally fortified with vitamin A and vitamin D.

MOLASSES

Residue left after repeated crystallization of sugar contains sucrose, glucose and fructose.

Contents per 100gm are

Sucrose	67%
Iron	500mg
Calories	260

MUSHROOM

It is agricus compestris.

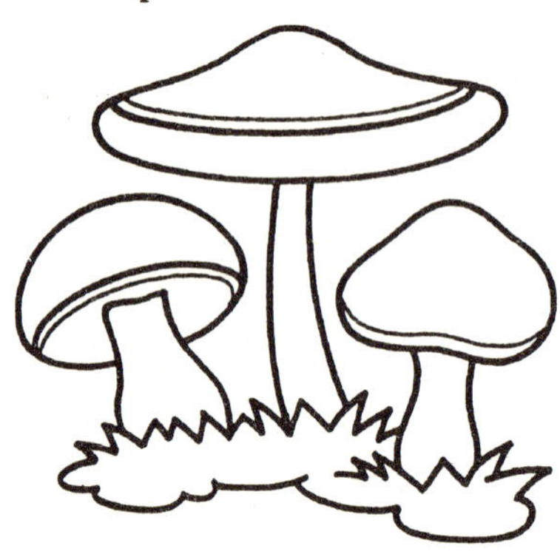

Contents per 100gram are

Proteins	11.9gm	Iron	1.4mg
Fat	21.1gm	Calories	241
Calcium	7mg		

OLIVE

Friuts of evergreen tree. Olive oil is used in cooking as salad oil. It contains a very little polyunsaturated fatty acid.

Content per 100 gram are

Protein	0.9gm	Iron	1mg
Fat	11gram	Calories	116
Calcium	60mg		

ORANGE

Fruits of citrus sinesis. Nutritive value due to vitamin C content.

Contents per 100gm are

Carbohydrate	8.5mg
Protein	0.6mg
Calcium	40mg
Iron	0.3mg
Carotene	50ug
Vitamin C	40 – 60mg
Calories	32

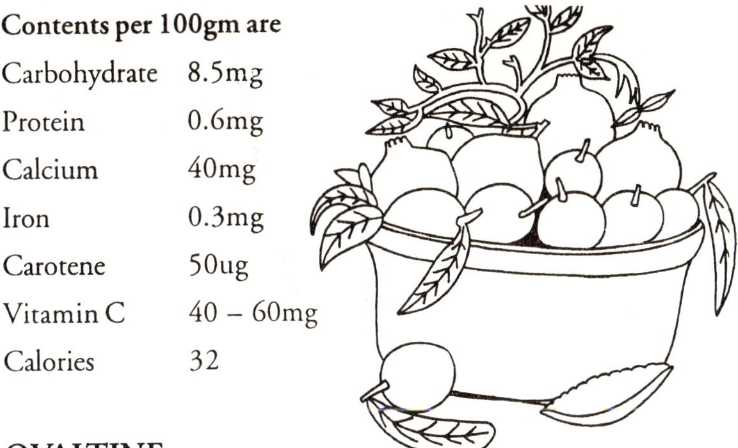

OVALTINE

It is a preparation of malt extract, milk, eggs, coca and soya, to be taken as beverage when added to milk. It is fortified with Vitamin B1, D and nicotinic acid.

PALM OIL

It is an oil extract from pericarp or pulp beneath the outer skin. It is reddish due to high content of alpha carotene and betacarotene.

It contains only 5 – 12% polyunsaturated fatty acid – linoleic acid.

PAPAYA

Large green fruit of carica papaya. It is arich source of vitamin A&C

Contents per 100gm are

Water	89gm
Carbohydrates	9gm
Carotene	800µg
Vitamin C	80mg

Proteolytic enzyme papain is obtained from the skin of the fruit. It is used in tendering meat. Rate of reaction is slow at room temperature and maximum activity is at 80°C.

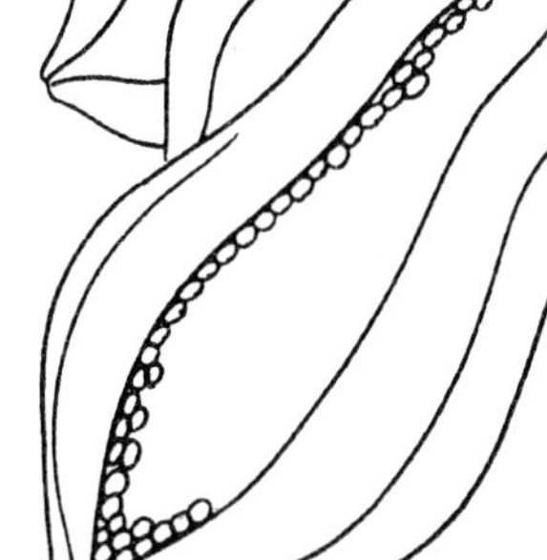

PEAS

Seeds of pisum sativum.

Contents per 100 gram are

Sugar	4gm	Iron	2mg
Starch	7gm	Carotene	300µg
Fiber	5gm	Vitamin C	15 – 35mg
Protein	6gm	Calories	80

GROUNDNUTS

Seeds of legume arachis hypogaea. It is a source of protein in many tropical diets. Oil is used for cooking. Residue after oil extraction is a valuable sources of proteins for animal feed.

Content per 100 gram are

Protein	25gm	B1	0.84mg
Fat	43gm	B2	0.12mg
Iron	1.9mg	Nicotinic acid	16mg

Peanut butter is also available.

PICKLES

Vegetable immersed in 5 – 10% brine and undergo lactic acid fermentation while the salts prevent the growth of undesirables. The sugars in vegetables are broken down to lactic acid at 25 degree C and process takes a few weeks. It finishes at 1% acidity.

SWEET POTATO

Tubers of herbaceous. Flesh may be white, yellow or pink.

Contents per 100 gram are

Protein	22 gram	Iron	0.8mg
Fat	1.1gm	Carotine	150µg
Calories	9%	Vitamin C	19mg

SMOKE POINT

Term is used with references to frying oils. Temperature at which the decomposition product become visible (bluish smoke); the temperature varies with different fats and ranges between 160 and 260 degree centigrade.

SOFT DRINKS

It is sweetened or unsweetened water charged with CO2 and O2 under pressure. The principal ingredients of soft drinks are carbon dioxide, sugars, citric acid, colouring and flavouring agents

Fruits juices are non-carbonated drinks, orange, juice contains vitamin C while mango juice is nutritionally very rich due to addition of milk.

SWEETENING AGENTS

There are three types of agent

- Sugars of which commonest is sucrose, fructose has 173% sweetness of sucrose, glucose 74% maltase 33%, Lactose 16%.
- Synthetic nonnutritive sweetners as saccharine (550 times sweet as sucrose).
- Various other chemicals such as glycerol and glycine (70% sweet as sucrose).

TEA

Nutritive value of coffee, tea & cocoa

Nutrition	Coffee	Tea	Cocoa
Proteins	1.8	0.9	7.2
Fat	2.2	1.1	8.8
Carbohydrate	13.8	16.4	16.2
Calcium	0.680	0.034	0.27
Phosphorus	0.050	0.032	0.20
Vit 'A'	102	51	408
Calories	98	60	213

TOFFEE

A sweet meat that is essentially a dispersion of minute globules of fat in a super saturated sugar solution made from fat, milk, sugar and confectioners glucose. Toffees are boiled at a high temperature of 260degree. to 270degree. C.

Contents per 100gm are

Water	4 – 8gm	Calories	435
Sugars	70gm	Calcium	95mg
Protein	2gm	Iron	1.5mg
Fat	17gm		

TOMATO

Fruit of lycopersicon esculentum; contents per 100gm are

Proteins	1.1gm	Iron	0.6mg
Carbohydrates	3gm	Nicotinic Acid	200µgm
Calories	19	Vitamin C	2.3mg
Calcium	11mg		

VANILLA

Extract of vanilla, bean, fruit, and orchid. Arachs aromaticus and related species. Fruits are allowed to ferment, crushed and extracted with alcohol. Chief flavouring principal is vanillin. Vanilla sugar is ground bean mixed with sugar.

VINEGAR

It is a product of a double fermentation. It contains 5% acitic acid with flavours derived from esters and a higher alcohols. It is used in salad as an preservative.

WHEY

It is the residue from milk after removal of casein and most of fat; also known ac lacto serum. It contains about 1% protein together with all lactose and minerals. 92% is water. Whey cheese can be made by heat coagulation of protein and whey butter from small amount (0.25%) fat.

WINE

Fermented grape juice containing 9 –10% ethyl alcohol. Beverages made by fermenting other food, juices and sugar in the presence of leaves, vegetables or roots are called wines. Fortified wines as Madeira, Sherry and Port have added spirit to bring the alcohol content to 15%.

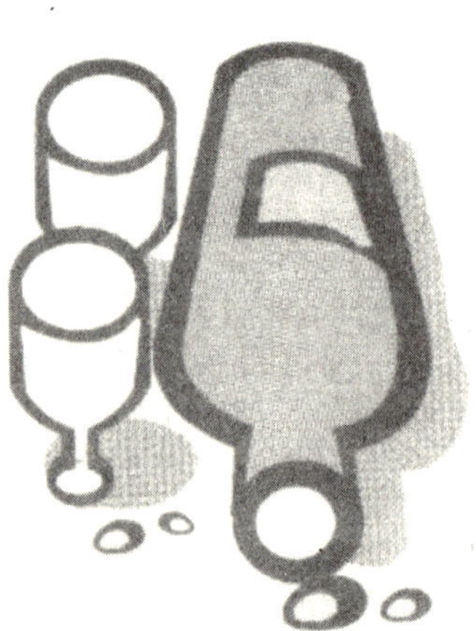

YEAST

These are grouped as fungi although they are unicellular. It is used in brewing, wine making and baking. Varities such as candida utilities are grown on carbohydrate or hydrocarbon media as animal feed and potential human feed. 50% is protein by dry weight.

ZAMUN

This fruit reduces the blood sugar. Its seed contains glucoside 'Jamboline' and flagie acid which are reputed to have the ability to check the conversion of starch into sugar in case of excess production of glucose. Jamun seeds are powdered and given to diabetics.

CHOCOLATE AND CONFECTIONERY

By weight chocolate and confectionery is at least half sugar. Which is unsuitable for diabetes, weight reducers and for teeth. Chocolate made from cocoa, sugar, cocoa butter and flavourings contains about 40% fat. Pastery, fruit gums, chocolate and liquorice contain mineral and small amounts of protein. Toffee and fudge contain added salt and should be avoided in case of hypertension.

CHEESE

Most cheeses are excellent sources of protein, calcium and phosphorus. They are good source of riboflavin and supply B vitamins but are lacking in vitamin 'C'. These are good sources of vitamin A, D and E. All these are poor source of iron.

Cheese is virtually carbohydrate free, most cheese is high in fat. It contains cholesterol and a high proportion of saturated fatty acids. Some cottage and curd cheeses are made out of skin milk are lower in content. Cream cheese is highest in energy. Cheddar contains are best sources of calcium. Soft cheeses like cottage are low in calcium. Processed cheese are slightly lower in protein and higher water contents.

Nutrients per 25 gms. Of confectionery

Nutrient	Camembert	Chdddar	Cheshire	Edam	Gorgonzola	Processed	Spread	Stilton	Cottage
Protein (grams)	6	6½	6½	6	6½	5¼	4½	6½	4
Fat (grams	6	8¾	7½	5¾	7¾	7½	5¾	10	1[a]
Cholesterol (milligrams)	20	25 —	25	—	20	—	—	3.5	
Calcium (milligrams)	40	200	155	185	135	180	125	90	20
Phosphorus (milligrams)	70	135	115	130	95	120	110	75	—
Sodium (milligrams)	350	155	175	245	305	230	290	290	80
Potassium (milligrams)	30	30	25	40	45	20	40	40	—
Magnesium (milligrams)	5	10	5	5	10	10	5	5	—
B vitamins: riboflavin (milligrams)	0.2	0.13	0.13	01	—	0.1	—	0.08	0.07
Vitamin E (a tocopherol milligrams)	—	0.25	—	—	—	—	—	—	—
Vitamin A (microgram equivalents)	60	105	90	70	90	90	70	120	7
Vitamin D (micrograms)	0.05	0.09	0.08	0.06	0.08	0.08	0.06	0.1	0.005
Vitamin C	0	0	0	0	0	0	0	0	0

GOOSE BERRY — It is an edible fruit.

It contains per 100 gram

Carbohydrate	9 grams	Carotene	600 microgram
Protein	2 grams	Vitamin 'C'	30 mg
Calories	48		

ICE CREAMS

Per 60 gram containing 10% fat

Energy	11.5	Carbohydrate	12 gm
Protein	2.5 gram	Calcium	80 mg
Fat	6.5 gram	Phosphorus	60 mgm
Cholesterol	25 mgm	Iron	0.15 mgm

Vitamin A,D, C are Nil

Sugar is the main agent for promoting growth of bacteria when taken in sticky form. Acidity at which enamel begins to be dissolved reaches within 5 minutes of eating sugar. Alkalinity of saliva protects it. Very acid foods are capable of dissolving away the enamel. Front teeth are particularly affected hence acid cola should be taken with a strew.

IODINE VALUE — It is a measure of degree of unsaturation of a fat by the extent of uptake of iodine i.e. grams iodine per 100 gram of fat.

Iodine values are

Butter	22-38
Lard	54-70

Nutritive values of 25 gram cheese

Nutrient	Camembert	Chdddar	Cheshire	Edam	Gorgonzola	Processed	Spread	Stilton	Cottage
Protein (grams)	6	6½	6½	6	6½	5¼	4½	6½	4
Fat (grams	6	8¾	7½	5¾	7¾	7½	5¾	10	1[a]
Cholesterol (milligrams)	20	25 —	25	—	20	—	—	3.5	
Calcium (milligrams)	40	200	155	185	135	180	125	90	20
Phosphorus (milligrams)	70	135	115	130	95	120	110	75	—
Sodium (milligrams)	350	155	175	245	305	230	290	290	80
Potassium (milligrams)	30	30	25	40	45	20	40	40	—
Magnesium (milligrams)	5	10	5	5	10	10	5	5	—
B vitamins: riboflavin (milligrams)	0.2	0.13	0.13	01	—	0.1	—	0.08	0.07
Vitamin A (microgram equivalents)	60	105	90	70	90	90	70	120	7
Vitamin D (micrograms)	0.05	0.09	0.08	0.06	0.08	0.08	0.06	0.1	0.005

Some cottage cheese, made from skim milk, is fat free

Coconut oil	8-10
Cotton seed	104-114
Linseed	170-202

GOURDS — (cucumber, pumpkin, squash, bottle gourd)

All contains more than 90% water

Protein	1%
Vitamin 'C'	10 mg

yellow pumpkin contains 900 microgram carotene.

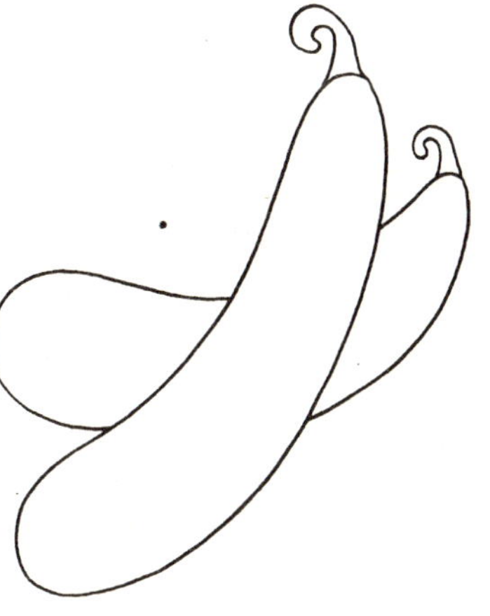

CHOLESTEROL — It is a part of body structure and a normal constituent of blood stream. Most adults contains 150 grams. It is needed for cell membrane, particularly nerves and also for the synthesis of some hormones. Bile salts and vitamins D. Animal foods contains cholesterol but it is not an essential nutrient. Body synthesizes double the amount of cholesterol eaten from outside. Food containing the most cholesterol are brain and egg yolk. Plant foods don't contain cholesterol.

Lean meats contain high percentage of cholesterol.

Cholesterol free foods include — egg white, all plant foods like oils, fruits, nuts, vegetables, cereals, cooking fats and margarine made entirely from plant oils and fats, jams, sweets.

Malnutrition

What do you understand by malnutrition?

Malnutrition may be due to improper or inadequate food intake. It may also result from inadequate absorption of food. Deficient supply of food, poor dietary habbits, food faddism and emotional factors may also limit food intake. Certain metabolic abnormalities may also result it.

MARASMUS

What is Marasmus?

Clinical picture of marasmus is due to general starvation. It may be the result of inadequate calorie intake or due to improper feeding habits.

What are the clinical features of marasmus?

There is a failure to gain weight followed by loss of weight until obvious emaciation results. Skin becomes wrinkled due to loose subcutaneous fat. Fat becomes shrunken and child looks wizened like a monkey face. Abdomen may be distended. Appetite may be increased or reduced with occasional diarrhea. There may be associated vitamin deficiency.

KWASHIORKOR

What is Kwashiorkor?

Cicely Williams described this in 1933. The child becomes apathetic, anemic, anorexic and oedematous. He develops diarrhea.

There is severe growth retardation. Child looses weight but due to oedema he does not look like skinny. There may be pleural effusion (water in lungs) and ascites (water in abdomen)

What type of skin changes takes place in kwashiorkor?.

Skin changes may involve any part of the body specially lower limbs. Darkening of skin appears in areas of irritation but not in those exposed to sunlight. There may be areas of pigmentation and depigmentation. Cracks appear at folds and ulcer may develop. Hair becomes brown and depigmented and coarse.

What is the difference between Marasmus and Kwashiorkor?

Difference between Marasmus and Kwashiorkor

Feature	Marasmus	Kwashiorkor
Cause	Deficiency of calories	Protein deficiency
Washing	Thin, lean and skiny	Flabby child. Moon face
Muscle wasting	Severe	Lesser
Loss of weight	Severe	Masked by oedema
Mental changes	Abscent	Present
Skin changes	None	Pigmentation
Hair changes	Slight change in texture	Often sparse, brownish
Hepatic enlargement	None	Frequent

What is protein calorie malnutrition?

This is a super imposition of marasmus + kwashiorkor.

Wellcome classification of PCM

Weight % of Harvard standard	Odema	
	Present	Abscent
80 to 60	Kwashiorkor	Under nutrition
Below 60	Marasmus	Kwashiorkor

What is the cheapest and best treatment of PCM?

National institute of nutrition has formulated an energy protein mixture

Whole wheat roasted	40 gm
Ground nut roasted	10gm
Bengal gram roasted	16 gm
Jaggery roasted	20 gm
Total weight	86 gm
Energy	330 Kcl
Protein	11.3 gm

Giving this mixture for 3 months help the child.

OBESITY

Obesity is the bank balance of calories. If your weight is 10 % more than expected weight you are over weight but if it is 20 % more than you are an obese. If you spend less calories than your consumption then you will gain weight.

What are sedentary activities?

Reading, writing, eating, watching TV, sewing, playing cards, typing, office work and activities done sitting are sedentary activities and you loose about 80 / 100 calories per hour.

What are light activities?

Cooking food, doing dishes, dusting hand washing, ironing, walking, work done while standing requiring arm movements are light activities and one spends 110 to 160 calories/hour.

What are moderately active activities?

Mopping and scrubbing, sweeping, polishing/ waxing, laundering, carpentry work and walking moderately fast are moderate activities. It requires 170 – 240 calories/ hour.

What about vigorous activities?

Heavy scrubbing and waxing, fast walking, bowling, golfing, doing physical activity are vigorous activities and require 250 – 350 calories per hour.

What about strenuous activities?

Swimming, playing tennis, running, cycling, dancing and playing foot ball are strenuous activities. It requires 350 – 900 calories / hour.

What are the important causes of obesity?

(1) Parentral nutrition – It may activate genetic tendency towards over weight. When one parent is over weight there are 50 % chances that child will be obese. Chances increase to 80 % when both parents are obese.

(2) Infant overfeeding – Pattern can be established in infancy. Overfeeding an infant produces a fat baby who becomes a plump child and an obsese adolescent.

(3) Breast feeding – Chances of breast fed child becoming obese are rare.

(4) Recent investigations have shown that in every obese person number and size of adipose cells are greater.

(5) Increased appetite – Obesity is invariably caused by a greater intake of calories in food than expenditure of calories. This disproportion results from an appetite for food that is greater than required to maintain normal weight.

(6) Satiety level – Appetite is a desire for food and satiety is a lack of desire to eat more. The inability to reach the point of

satiety may be the variable that differentiates the obese from the normal weight person.

(7) Habitual over- eating - Repeated over feeding beyond satiety results in the setting of the appestat at a level so high that satisfaction can no longer be obtained by normal food intake. When appestat is conditioned or set at a higher level the person is not conscious of over eating.

(8) Effect of environment – Habitual over eating may come solely from environment. In a house where a laden table is regularly set and where the quantity and quality of food are over emphasized by parents, it is common.

What is the standard weight for height in males?

Weight for height in males

Height cms	Weight kg	Over weight Limit (+20%)	Under weight Limit (-20%)
148	47.5	57	38
152	49.0	59	39
156	51.5	62	41
160	53.5	64	43
164	56.0	67	45
172	62.0	74.6	49.5
176	65.6	78.5	52.4
180	68.5	82	56.5

What is the standard weight for height in females?

Weight for height in females

Height cms kg	Weight kg	Over weight Limit (+20%)	Under weight Limit (-20%)
148		46.5	56.0 37.0
152		48.5	58 39.0
156		50.5	60.5 40.5
160		52.5	63.5 42.0
164		55.5	66.0 44.0
168		58.5	69.0 46.5
172		60.5	72.5 48.5
176		64.0	77.0 51.0

Can psychological problems also lead to obesity?

Yes, for many people psychological problems act as a sedative to give temporary solace just as alcohol does to others. These are people who lack in any other interest in life. They live only to eat.

Often the mothers of obese children are themselves emotionally starved and disappointed from their husband. In compensation they pour out the children the love they would have given to their husband.

What is Broca's index?

It is the way to know the expected weight of body. According to Brocas index.

Standard weight in kg = Height in centimeter minus 100.

But this formula does not take body build into consideration.

How Ponderal index helps?

$$\text{Ponderal index} = \frac{\text{Height in inches}}{\text{Under root weight in pound.}}$$

This depends on both height and weight and is considered as an index of obesity.

What is mid triceps skin fold?

It is a rapid and precise method. A triceps skin fold thickness of 12m.m. or supra iliac fold of 8m.m. or more suggest obesity in man, twice in case of a woman.

What are the effects of obesity?

The desire to be attractive is the most frequent reason why over weight people want to reduce. The constant fear of embarrassment and humiliation is so great that they often remain depressed.

What is the relation of longevity and obesity?

Death from degenerative complications are higher in obese people. It is 70% higher. Death rate is 15% higher in obese people at any age.

How obesity is related to cardiovascular system?

Obesity is the most common agent in causing arteriosclerotic cardiovascular disease and high blood pressure. Obesity also helps in precipitating the symptoms of angina pectoris. Obese person is able to get less air into lungs even after forcible inhalations.

Can obesity result in early diabetes?

Insurance figures show 8% more deaths in a patient of diabetes + obesity. Central obesity is worst. Otherwise also obese people are exposed to increased risk of hernias, cholecystitis and osteoarthritis. Infertility is also more common in obese people.

MANAGEMENT OF OBESE PEOPLE

What are the common methods of reducing?

Common methods are

1. Reduced food intake
2. Regulated physical exercise
3. Medicines if any.

How reduced food intake helps?

Obesity is seen as a consequence of positive balance of energy consumed over energy expanded. So reduction in amount of food will reduce obesity.

It takes about 3500 extra calories to produce a pound of store fat. For each pound to be gained or lost there must be 3500 calories more or less in diet. To loose 2 pounds one has to consume 1000 calories less for a week.

What is ketogenic diet?

It is a low calories diet which contains 70% fat calories, 20% from protein and 10% from carbohydrate.

Can keeping a 'fast' help in reducing weight?

Yes keeping fast 2 to 14 days encourages weight loss and produces post fast loss of appetite. Subjects who are having water retention gives better results specially females. Obesity is never resistant to a low calories and dieting.

Can low calories food help?

Yes, very much. One should consume lot of leafy vegetables, cabbage, spinach, lettuce etc. And one should learn to avoid butter, egg, fried food and sweets.

Salad consumption help in reducing weight.

How regulated physical exercise help?

A slow walk for half an hour will result in an extra expenditure of 50 calories. Heavy exercises in reducing weight defeats its purpose because in return it increases its appetite.

Can spot reducing is possible?

Spot reducing means to loose weight only from one part of body which is not possible. There is no known method that will weigh off one area and not other.

What type of exercises help in loosing weight?

Expenditure of calories per hour.

Activity	Calories	Activity	Calories
Dressing	33	Mental work	7 to 8
Sitting at rest	15	Sawing wood	420
Walking	130–200	Cycling	180–300
Running	500–900	Swimming	200–700
Sewing	25–30	Climbing	200–900
Sweeping	110	Wrestling	900
Knitting	31	Scrubbing floor	261

Can drugs help in reducing weight?

No drug is very safe and reliable in reducing weight. Extract of thyroid was in use in past. Now amphetamines have been used in management by increasing B.M.R. and diuresis. Phentermine a nonamphetamine in a single daily dose of one capsule reduces appetite.

What are your suggestions to weight reducers?

1. Persons who are overweight should reduce and those who are little overweight need not to reduce. They should watch

their diet to not to put on more weight.

2. Take it easy. Loss of pound or two per week is enough.
3. Plan meals around familiar foods. Select food which gives you satisfaction. It is important to establish patterns of eating that can be followed for a longer time. Undesirable and unattractive combinations prove disastrous.
4. Many reducing diets which include only a few foods may have inadequate nutrients.
5. Choose a variety of foods of lower calories.
6. Budget your calories to take care of your special occasions such as holidays and parties. Keep busy so that you are not tempted to eat food off and on.
7. Take advantage to increase the physical activity.

Approximate value of common food

	No.	Weight gm	Calories	Protein	Fats
Chapaties	2	57	193	5	5.5
Rice	1 plate	100	110	6	0.2
Pulse	1 cup	150	284	16.0	9.0
Omelette	1	39	77	5.8	5.7
Bread	2 slice	46	120	4.0	1.0
Biscuits	2	16	64	1.6	2.0
Milk	1 cup	702	300	9.0	6.0
Apple	1	66	42	0.2	0.3
Orange	1 glass	602	70	0.1	
Sugar	1 tea spoon	5	20		
Ground nut		28	155	7.6	11.3
Butter	1 table spoon	14	126		14
Ghee	1 table spoon	15	135		15

Toxins of Food

EPIDEMIC DROPSY

In 1926 Sarkar found that the contamination of mustard oil with argemone oil is cause of epidemic dropsy. The mustard oil being of pungent odour is capable of hiding the odour of Argemone seed oil.

What is the pathology of epidemic dropsy?

Toxic factor of yellow Mexican poppy is alkaloid sanguinarine'.oxidation of pyruvate to lactate is stopped with resultant stimulation of pyruvate in tissues and blood. Blood vessels dilate resulting in oedema putting strain on heart.

What are its clinical features?

First patient feels loss of appetite, nausea and diarrhoea. Later on patient develops swelling over feet specially after walking. Oedema is pitting but tender and hot. In certain cases there may be pleural and cardiac effusion. There may be mild fever. Patient may die.

Is there any prevention?

- The contamination can be brought down to negligible levels during the refining process of oil by passing live steam into it for 30 minutes.
- Toxicity tends to wane off on keeping the oil for some months or heating at 240 degree 'C' for 15 minutes.

LATHYRISM

Hippocrates stated that men and women who ate peas continuously became impotent in legs. Toxin B oxalye amino – L

– alamine (BOAA) present in pulse of 'Khesari Dal' produces the toxic effect upon the nervous system.

How is the mode of onset of disease?

In 50 % cases onset is sudden and severe. Person working in field may fall down. There is dull aching with increasing stiffness of lower limbs.

What is its warning stage?

There will be sudden agonizing pain in calf or back of things with a spasmodic contraction of these muscles. If person stops eating Khasari Dal disease does not progresses.

What are different stages of the disease?

There are four stages

(1) First stage (Non stick stage) Patient walks with short steps and jerky movements. Heels don't rest on the ground. There is marked swaying of hips and head to counter balance.

(2) Second stage (One stick stage) There is flexion of knee and crossing of gait. Person walks on his toes with muscular rigidity. Patient needs one stick to support.

(3) Third stage (Two stick stage) Symptoms are more severe. Gait is slow and clumpsy and patient gets tired soon. Patient can walk with the help of two sticks.

(4) Crawler stage – Knees become completely bent and patient crawls on his knees and palm.

What is the simple method of removal of toxin?

Lathyrus seeds are soaked in boiling water for one hour. 90 to 95 % of toxin will drain water with water soluble vitamins.

On large scale, parboiling of water will help.

EPIDEMIC GOITRE

In India 120 million people live in known goiter epidemic areas and about 40 million suffer from it.

What do you understand by Goitre?

Goitre indicates enlargement of thyroid gland situated in front and lower part of neck. When goiter is found in more than 10 % people it is referred as an endemic goiter.

What is the cause?

Daily requirement of iodine is 100 to 150 mcg for adults and 90 % of it comes through food and water. Milk, meat, cereals, vegetables are rich in iodine. Lack of iodine causes it .

What are the sign and symptoms?

There is soft, diffuse and symmetrical enlargement of gland, gradually swelling becomes asymmetrical, nodular and firm. Enlarged gland may press esophagus and laryngeal nerve. Pulse becomes fast and tremors develop. Consumption of iodine salt helps.

ENDEMIC FLUOROSIS

This is caused by excess intake of fluoride and changes in teeth and bone develops. Sorghum based diets have been found retaining more of fluoride.

What is dental fluorosis?

It is the earliest and most sensitive index of fluoride over intake during the period of teeth eruption. Upper incisors are first to be affected. Enamel looses shining and lusture and become discoloured and pitted. White opacities are seen.

What happens in skeletal fluorosis?

Patient develops pain, numbness and tingling sensation. Person complaints of small joints pain. Bones may become marble white. A concentration of 0.5 to 1 ppm protects against dental caries.

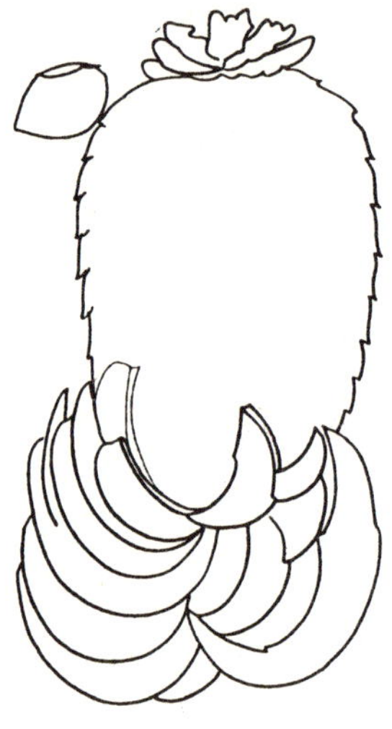

Feeding of Different Groups

INFANT FEEDING

The main food of most infants is breast milk which is a nature's gift to human kind – a complete food.

What is colostrum?

The yellowish secretion from the breast in the first few days is called colostrum. It has a high protein and vitamin 'A' confers immunity against certain infections. It also helps in development of enzymes required for digestion.

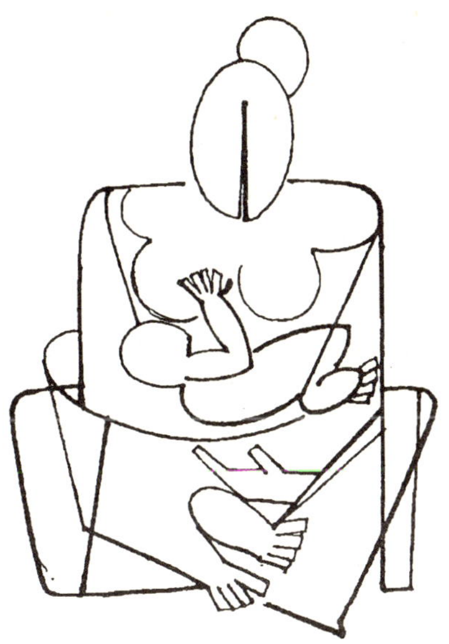

When onset of lactation starts?

The onset of milk starts about 3rd day after delivery. After birth baby should suckle the breast as soon as after birth because it increases milk secretion and helps uterus to contract. During early month he will require 8 – 10 feeds. After second month 5 – 6 feeds will be sufficient and child will sleep well. For first 3 – 4- months breast feeding meets the requirement of child in full. Whether the lady is rich or poor, quality of milk remains the same.

What are the restrictions of breast feeding?

- Markedly inverted nipples, fissures and cracks of nipples may not allow mother to feed children.
- Septicaemia, eclampsia, active TB, typhoid and severe neurosis are absolute contraindications to breast feeding.

How will you recognize under feeding?

Symptoms of under feeding will be –

(1) Crying – Child may suckle for a long time, will fall deeply asleep at the end of feed and wake up crying more after an hour. He may again suck for a short time and then start to scream.

(2) Failure to gain weight – Baby should gain 30 gram of weight daily about 150 – 250 gram weekly. So long he is gaining weight need not to worry.

(3) Constipation – Underfed babies may develop constipation. Hunger stools are small dark greenish mucous stool.

What are the disadvantages of bottle feeding?

It has increased the sickness & mortality due to-

- Lack of sufficient sanitary preparations of bottles and milk formula.
- Ignorance of basic rules of sanitation.
- Lack of facilities for making formula and lack of refrigeration.

What do you understand by weaning?

It is the process in which an infant's diet pattern is gradually changed to semi solids from liquid milk. Solids can be added from fourth month but weaning should start after six months. After this breast milk alone can not sustain the growth. Semisolid foods in the shape of gruel or paste, khichdi, and suji halwa may be given. Feeding schedule should be flexible and not tight. It should be based on signs of hunger rather than fixed hour of feeding.

What important points are to be remembered about feeding an infant?

- Rigid adherence to clock schedules by over enthusiastic mother may contribute to the baby's confusion.
- The infant should empty at least one breast at each feeding to stimulate for refill.
- If mother is doctor or so in that case after 6 – 8 weeks supplementary replacement feeding of cow's or powdered milk has the advantage permitting the mother to perform her official duties but she should not hesitate to breast feed when she is available at home.
- Mother should know that only hungry child will search for nipple.
- Regurgitation and vomiting are frequent signs of over feeding.

What should be the food for toddlers?

During this period child shows a marked decrease in appetitute during the second year because the child grows at a slower rate in comparison to first year.

Children can share family food by the age of two. He may be given kheer, custard or ice creams. Fruits are ideal snacks.

NUTRITION DURING PREGNANCY AND LACTATION

Nutrition needs during pregnancy include the normal requirement of mother and those of the developing fetus including uterus and placenta.

What is the energy requirement during pregnancy?

Additional need of calories is small during first half of pregnancy while an increase of 300 calories per day is estimated for the second half of pregnancy. Young active lady will require more.

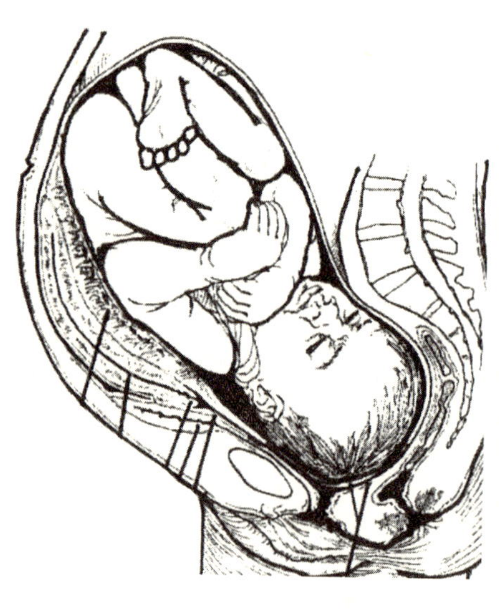

During lactation 130 calories is required for each 100 ml of milk. For total 600 ml of milk about 800 – 1000 extra calories will be required. About 2gm. of food protein are required during lactation to produce 1gm. of milk protein.

What will be the requirement of iron?

From 700 – 1000 mg of iron must be absorbed and utilized by the mother throughout the span of pregnancy. Out of it 240 mg iron is saved due to cessation of menstrual flow. Daily increase of 8 to 10 mg will provide sufficient iron. Rate of absorption increases during third trimester.

What will be the requirement of calcium?

An increased retention of calcium is required both for fetal bones, teeth and maternal skeleton during lactation, 1.5 gram of calcium is needed during pregnancy while demand increases to 2 gram during lactation. High doses of vitamin 'D' of 400 i.u will be needed for the utilization of calcium and phosphorus by fetus and mother.

NUTRITION AFTER FIFTY

Requirement decreases due to physiological, psychological and social problems.

What physiological changes occur during old age?

- Loss of teeth interfere with proper mastication. Inability to chew food will reduce tolerance of certain type of food. Hard solid foods are avoided.
- Secretion of digestive enzymes by stomach, pancreas and intestine diminish. Therefore ability to digest food is diminished.
- Changes in intestinal mucosa may impede absorption of nutrition.
- Transportation of food

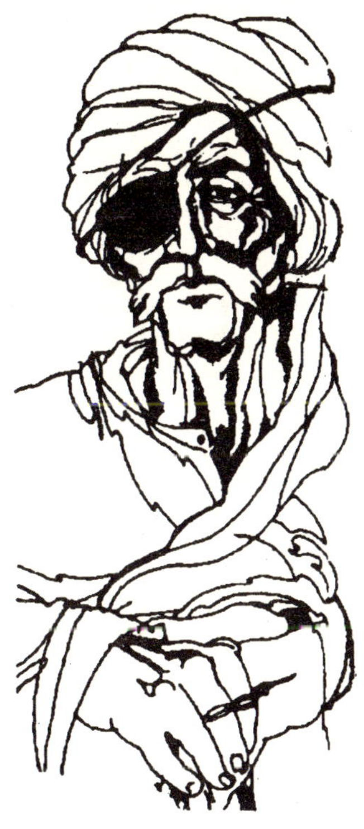

nutrients from intestinal tract to different tissues is affected by change in circulation and reduced O2 uptake.

- The basal metabolism decreases with advancing age and total energy requirement also decreases.
- As a result of psychological changes person develops likes and dislikes for different foods.
- The sense of taste and smell are less acute in later life thus interferes with appetite for many foods.
- Sometimes the frustration and isolation from the people and feeling of being rejected and unwanted may be expressed as complaints against food.

Loss of calcium may lead to osteoporosis. Calories requirement may be reduced by 10 % per every decade. Fats should be limited to 50 gm / day.

What is the balanced diet for an old person?

Balanced diet for old person

Food stuff	Man		Woman	
	Veg	Non veg	Veg	Non veg
Cereals (gm)	280	200	200	200
Pulses (gm)	85	55	85	55
Meat / fish (gm)		55		55
Egg (gm)		30		30
Green leafy vegetables	85	85	85	85
Roots / Tubers	55	55	55	55
Other vegetables	55	55	55	55
Fruits (gm)	55	55	30	30
Vegetable oil	30	30	30	30
Sugar (gm)	30	30	30	30

Describe the nutritional requirement of old age.

Nutritional requirement of an old age

Nutrient	Man	Woman
Calories	2000	1700
Protein (gm)	70	60
Calcium (gm)	0.8	0.8
Iron (mg)	20	20
Vit – A (i.u.)	5000	5000
Thiamine (mg)	1.2	1.0
Riboflavin (mg)	1.4	1.2
Nicotinic acid (mg)	12	10
Vitamin – C (mg)	50	50
Vitamin – D (i.u.)	400	400

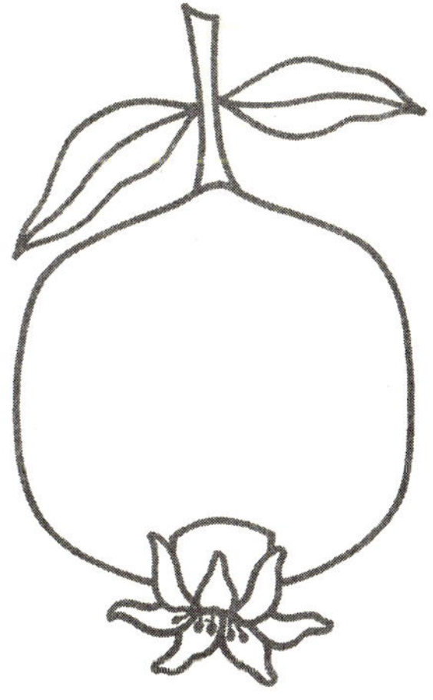

Nutrition for Sports Man

Who is a reference sports man?

Reference sportsman is defined as one aged 20 – 39 years weighing 60 kg in body weight and having 7 – 15 % body fat. Daily he involves 4 hours in moderate activity during practice. He needs 3600 Kcal of energy which can be obtained at ration level giving 4320 Kcal. 20 % is lost during processing, kitchen and wastage.

Who is a reference sports woman?

Reference woman is 20 – 39 years of age and weighing 50 kgs. She spends 4 hours in moderate activity. She requires 2900 Kcal i.e. 3500 Kcal at ration level.

Carbohydrate can provide energy up to 55 – 64 % of total requirement. Protein can supply about 12 – 14 % of energy and upper limit can be 2gm. per kg.

What is the recommended dietary intake of nutrients at ration level?

Nutrition at ration level

	Reference Sports Man	Reference Sports Woman
Net calories	4320	3480
Proteins (gm)	100–120	80–100
Calcium (gm)	1–2	1–2
Iron	50–75	60–100
Retinol	1000–2000	1000–2000
Thiamine (mg)	2–3	3–4
Vitamin – C (mg)	100–200	100–200
Nicotinic acid (mg)	40–50	40–50

What is the role of glycogen?

Ensure adequate glycogen stores to meet the needs of high intensity training period. Muscle and liver glycogen stores supply the glucose vital for production of anaerobic energy. It is necessary to replenish glycogen stores sfter long or intense training.

What is the balanced diet for sportsman in camps?

Balanced diet for sportsman in camps in grams

Food	Sports man		Sports woman	
	Veg	Non Veg	Veg	Non Veg
Rice	150	150	100	100
Wheat flour	250	250	200	200
White bread	150	150	100	100
Biscuits	20	20	20	20
Cheese / Paneer	50	-	30	-
Butter / Jam	20/50	20/50	20/50	20/50
Dal	35	-	35	-
Banana / apple	1	1	1	1
Orange	200	200	200	200
Root vegetables	150	150	100	100
Green leafy vegetables	175	175	150	150
Onion	100	100	50	50
Ghee	20	20	20	20
Vegetable oil	40	40	40	40
Sugar	50	50	40	40
Mutton / Chicken	-	250	-	200
Egg	100	-		50

What about fluids?

Many sportsman fail to hydrate adequately before events and fail to rehydrate afterwards. During games heavy sweating occurs at the expense of physical performance. Sweating may be as high as 2 litres per hour. Cold fluids 5 to 10^{0}C empty from the stomach faster than warmer one.

What is sports anemia?

The lower concentration of hemoglobin reflecting a beneficial increase in plasma volume and not a reduction in total hemoglobin.

What is carbohydrate loading?

From three days before 80 – 90 % carbohydrates are consumed till one hour before event. This way sufficient reserves are generated to meet the requirement of an event of 2 hours.

What should be the pre event meal?

Consumed a small meal of 500 to 1000 calories about 3 – 4 hours before an event so that it may not hamper digestion. For short events such as foot ball or short race a high carbohydrate meal, night before will help increase the glycogen in muscles.

What should be the post event meal?

Replacement of fluid and glycogen is important for a speedy recovery after an event. Drink water or dilute fluids frequently. It can take even 36 hours to rehydrate. A high carbohydrate diet replaces glycogen the fastest.

Different Aspects of Food

FOOD ADULTRATION

Adultration is the known process by which the quality or nature of a given substance is reduced by

- The removal of a vital element
- The addition of a foreign or an inferior substance.

What are the common types of adulterants?

- Incidental adulterants – These include pesticides, droppings of lizards and rodents.
- Intententional adulterants – These include sand, stone, mud, water to milk and mineral oil to edible oils.

What are common adulterants used?

Milk – Addition of plain contaminated water. Addition of starch, paper pulp are mixed to form a creamy layer.

Ghee – It is adulterated by vanaspati. To improve flavour tributyrin is added.

Pulses – Arhar pulse is adulterated with lathyrus. Metallic yellow is added to old stock to improve its colour and appearance.

Edible oil – Cheaper and mineral oils are added. Argemone oil is mixed with mustard oil resulting in dropsy. Dyes are added to improve the yellowish colour of oils.

Tea / Coffee – Tea is adulterated with exhausted tea leaves, saw dust. Coffee powder is adulterated with roasted dates, added colour and chicory.

Honey – It is mixed with sugar and jaggery solution and boiled with empty beehives.

FOOD FORTIFICATION

It is a process where by nutrients are added to foods to maintain or improve quality of food while enrichment is used for addition.

- Vanaspati ghee is fortified with vitamin 'A' and 'D' in the range of 2500 i.u and 175 i.u respectively per 100gm.
- Common salt is fortified with potassium iodate and supplied in endemic area.
- In certain countries sugar is fortified with vitamin 'A'
- Lysine is added to wheat flour while making modern bread.

FOOD ALLERGY

Allergy is a condition of exaggerated specific susceptibility to a substance which is harmless to a majority of population. Protein is the main factor for food allergy like milk, egg, fish etc. Skin lesions such as urticaria, rash and eczema are among most frequent symptoms of allergy. Nausea, vomiting and diarrhoea are common gastrointestinal symptoms.

FOOD POISONING

Food poisoning is characterized by gastroenteritis of abrupt nature due to ingestion of food / drink.

What is bacterial poisoning?

It is due to growth of bacteria salmonella group taken with the contaminated food like meat, fish, eggs and stale stored food. There will be pain, vomiting and diarrhoea after 8 hours.

Describe toxin type poisoning?

This is due to ingestion of certain substances formed as a result of multiplications of bacteria before ingestion. Cause may be

- Infected animal may be eaten
- Infected animal may excrete specific organism and contaminate food
- Human carrier of typhoid, infective hepatitis, worm infection may contaminate food by handling it.

How dangerous is botulism?

It is severe, neurologic and highly fatal. It is caused by ingestion of neurotoxin produced by growth of clostridium. It is common with tinned food. Symptoms develop with in 12 – 48 hours. There will be distorted diplopia (double vision) ptosis & difficulty in swallowing.

FOOD PRESERVATION

There is always a shortage of fresh food in developing countries.

Preservation helps in

- Making the seasonal vegetables available throughout the year
- Adding variety to the food preparation
- Saving time in procurement and cooking

How food is spoiled?

Undesirable changes takes place due to action of micro-organisms, moulds, yeasts and bacteria.

Mould growth on food looks like cottony appearance making food unfit for consumption. Moulds develop in warm, damp and dark places between 25 to 35^{0}C.

Where yeast grows?

Yeast grows usually on food such as fruits which contain water and sugar. The musty typical smell of spoiled grapes is due to growth of yeast. Yeast is reproduced by budding of cells. Yeast generally grows better in acid medium in presence of sufficient oxygen between 25 degree and 30 degree 'C. Yeast converts sugar of the fruit into alcohol and CO_2. Honey, jems, jellies are contaminated by yeast.

What are the principles of preservation?

Following are the common principles

(1) Asepsis – Nature has provided hard outer skin to keep the micro-organisms out of certain food articles such as banana, oranges, almonds, shell of egg etc.

(2) Filteration – The liquid food is filtered through a bacteria proof filter made of asbestos and unglazed porcelain. It is used as household filters for water.

(3) Blanching – To destroy enzymes to prevent decomposition, mild heat treatment is given to vegetables and fruits before canning or freezing.

(4) Prevention of oxidation – Oils, fats and sweets made of milk can become rancid on exposure to air. It can be prevented with antioxidants.

(5) Irradiation – It destroys micro-organisms. Ultraviolet lamps are used in sterilizing slicing knives in bakeries.

What are different methods of preservations?

(1) Bacteriostatic method –

In this micro-organisms are unable to grow in food i.e. dehydration, pickling, salting, smoking and freezing.

Dehydration is an unsuitable condition for micro-organisms because they need moisture to grow. Moisture can be removed by sunrays, heating and addition of suger and salt.

A layer of oil on top of any food prevents growth of micro-organisms.

At about 15^0 C potatoes, onions and apples can be stored for limited period. Chilling (0^0 C to 5^0C) preserves fruits / vegetables for 2 to 10 days.

(2) Bactericidal method –

In this procedures bacterias are killed i.e. canning, cooking and irradiation. Canning is done at temperature above 100^0C to kill organisms and to inactivate enzyme action. Temperature above 100^0C can be obtained by steam pressure sterilizers.

PARCHING

It is the process of puffing applied to cereals like wheat, rice and maize. Wet material is suddenly heated. Murmure and popcorn are examples of it. Starch present becomes more digestible after parching. Some loss of lysine aminoacid occur because of high temperature.

SPROUTING

Many cereals and dals can be sprouted to advantage. Vitamin 'C' content goes high may be even up to 10 times. Contents of thiamine, riboflavin and nicotine becomes double. Iron becomes free and more available to body.

FERMENTING

Making cured from milk is a good example of fermentation. For making idly and dosa rice mixture is to be fermented. It is done by micro-organisms. These multiply at right temperature. In making curd lactose is converted into lactic acid. Enzymes act on starch producing Co_2 producing bubbles. Fermented food are soft and spongy.

LIMEING

Lime can be incorporated into food item specially which are sour or acid type such as butter milk, rasam and fermented mixture used to make idli / dosa. It will cause destruction of thiamine and riboflavin.

COOKING

Each culture and religion has its own method of cooking, blending flavours.

How cooking helps?

Cooking improves the appearance of several foods and confers new flavours and makes food appetizing and palatable. Heat causes starch to swell and cell wall bursts and digestive enzymes can act upon. Cooking makes meat softer and worth being chewed. Bengal gram, soyabean and duck's egg contain trypsin inhibitors not allowing protein to be fully utilized, but cooking destroys trypsin inhibitors.

Which vegetables suffer more?

Root vegetables don't suffer much loss of nutrients by wet or dry cooking because the skin of vegetables prevent leaking out of nutrients. Hence potatoes, arvi should be boiled with skin. Losses due to leaching are less if vegetables are cut into bigger pieces. Losses are less if vegetables are just steamed.

All proteins are denatured and rhen coagulated by heat.

Coagulation occurs between 65^0 and 90^0 C.

There is generally no loss of minerals during cooking. Some being water soluble may be lost if cooking water is thrown out.

If tamarind with high acidity is added to cooking water it has a preservative effect on vitamins. It is preferable to cook leafy vegetables with the lid on withminimum exposure to air and minimum quantity of water.

Adding of soda destroys most of the thiamine.

PRESERVATIVES

Sulphur dioxide is the most commonly used preservative. It kills bacteria and is useful in fruits and vegetables because it prevents browning and preserves vitamins C. However it destroys thiamin and is only permitted is meat products. Benzoic acid is found naturally in loganberries and prunes. Proprionic acid and sorbic acid also occur naturally in food. They prevent growth of moulds. Nisin is an antibiotic found naturally in cheese and splits to aminoacids during digestion. Citrous fruits and bananas may have phenyls on the skin to prevent moulds. Common preservatives used are –

PHARMACOLOGICAL FOOD INTOLERANCE

What is pharmacological food intolerance?

Several different substances with pharmacological properties are present in food. Histamines and monoamines (tyramine and phenylethlamine) and methyl xanthines (caffeine, theophylline have pharmacological potential symptoms appearing on large consumption.

Food group	Food allowed to contain preservative	Permitted Preservative
Vegetables and fruits	Raw peeled potatoes or chips, any dehydrated vegetable, candied peel, dried fruit, jam Fruit juices, fruit pulp, tomato puree or pulp, pickles sauces Bananas or citrus fruit (on the skin)	Sulphur dioxide Sulphur dioxide or benozoic acid Phenyls
Dairy	All cheese Clotted cream Any cheese except cheddar, cheshire, soft cheese	Nisin and sorbic acid Nisin Nitrite
Flour	Bread Cakes, biscuits, pastry	Proprionic acid Proprionic acid or sorbic acid
Miscellaneous	Any canned food Gelatin, ginger, marzipan, caramel, vinegar, sugar, glucose syrup colours Flavours	Nisin Sulphur dioxide Benzoic acid or sorbic acid Sulphur dioxide or benzoic acid
Beverages	Beer, cider or perry Wine Soft drinks, glucose drinks Instant coffee or extract Drinking chocolate, tea extract	Sulphur dioxide Sulphur dioxide or sorbic acid Sulphur dioxide or benzoic acid Sulphur dioxide Benzoic acid

Can histamine produce food allergy?

Yes, histamine may result in reaction that is clinically similar to an IGE mediated food allergy. Elevated histamine levels correlate with migraine attacks. Foods with high content of histamine includes several cheeses, wines, several yeast products and several fishes. Improper refrigeration of these products results in dramatic rise in histamine content. Small amounts are present in liver, spinach and tomatoes.

How monoamines become intolerable?

These affect G.I. tract and CNS and have been associated with migraine headaches. Tyramine releases norephinephrine from tissue stores and results in rise of blood pressure. It is found in most aged cheese, brewer's yeast, pickled herrings.

Can salicyclates become intolerable?

Foods with high contents of natural salicylates include oranges, berries, pineapples, cucumbers, grapes, almond, peppermint, mint. 10 to 20% asthmatics react negatively to aspirin.

How methyl xanthines behave?

These are food in tea, coffee and chocolates. When consumed in large amount may cause hypertension. Caffeine stimulates gastric secretion and can cause esophageal reflex, nausea and diarrhoea.

TOLERANCE TO FOOD ADDITIVES

What is the role of nitrates?

Nitrates and nitrites are widely used as preservatives due to flavouring and colouring attributes, Nitrates may produce headache. Hot dogs, bacon, smoked fish have high concentration of it.

Can addition of sulphites be harmful?

It is naturally present in fermented food and often added to salad green, vegetables and fruits to maintain freshness. These are present in wines, beers and dry fruits. It mostly affects asthmatics.

How monosodium glutamate affects?

It is used an flavour enhancer in Asian Foods. In chinese restaurant syndrome symptoms occurs in 15-30 minutes and include headache, chest tightness, nausea and vomiting.

Can Tartrazine give adverse feeling?

It gives a lemon yellow colour to foods and some medicine. It is added to vitamin supplements, pickles, cakes, gelatins, packed soups, coloured candids, soft drinks, jillies and ice creams. Adverse reactions include bronchospasm and urticaria.

ANTIOXIDANTS

Antioxidant fight against harmful compounds produced during various activities. Different biochemical reactions in body continuously produce various free radicals. If these free radicals are not quenched by antioxidants, they cause damage to cells, protein, DNA and RNA resulting in various degenerative diseases such as cancer,arteriosclerosis and diabetes. Turmeric, garlic, cloves, selenium, vitamin E, vit. C are commonly used antioxidants.

DIFFERENT ASPECTS OF FOOD

What is the utility of having soup?

Soup is served at the beginning of formal dinners. They stimulate appetite and provide nourishment clear soups are ways to introduce fluids and contribute sodium chloride, potassium and other minerals. Milk / cream and nuts provide calories. Meat stock are rich in extractives, fully flavoured and stimulant to secretory cells of stomach. It should be taken 15- 20 minutes before actual dinner.

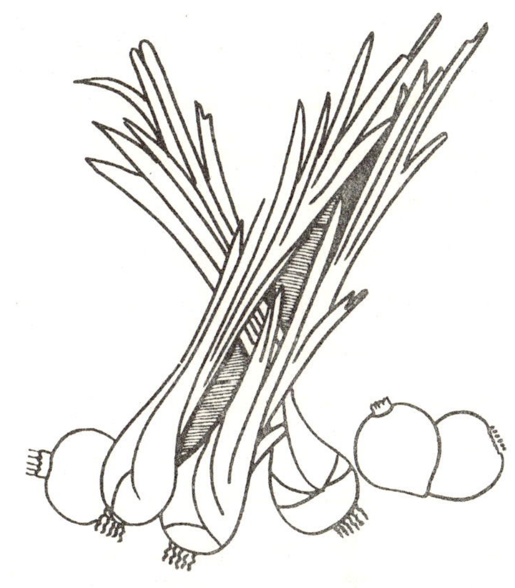

What is the role of salad?

It is always best to start a meal with fresh raw salad. Common vegetables used for salad are salad leaves, onions, cucumber, tomatoes, cabbage, carrots and turnip. All these vegetables should be thoroughly washed before cutting. Salad has minimum calories but provide roughage, minerals and vitamin 'C'.

Are condiments classified as food?

Condiments are not classified as food but are food adjuncts. Besides giving flavour and stimulating the flow of digestive juices these relieve flatulent – distension occurring from fermentation in intestine. Black pepper, cloves, chillies and coriander are all used in preparation of different dishes to give taste and flavour.

How is vinegar used?

Vinegar is a well known antiseptic and preservative. It is used for pickling fish, fruits and vegetables. It also softens hard muscle fibers of meat and cellulose of green vegetables. It is largely used in salads for preserving small onions.

How helpful is sweet dish / ice cream or puddings?

It is customary in formal dinners to serve soup in the beginning and sweet dish at last.

During process of eating food one looses certain amount of energy that is why certain people start sweating after food. To compensate it sweet is required which provides immediate calories.

What is the component of Betelnut?

Betelnut grows in bunches in yellow orange colour. Outer covering of fruit is removed from seed and is chopped into small pieces and boiled in water which makes nuts soft and reduces tannin content.

Constituents of arecanut / 100 gram

Proteins	5 – 9 gm
Carbohydrates	47 – 84 gram
Minerals	calcium, phosphorus, iron
Vitamins	carotene
Tanin	11- 26 mg
Alkaloids	150 – 670 mg

What is the composition of catechu?

Catechu or Kathha is the resinous extract obtained from acacia tree.

Composition of catechue is

Moisture	12.5 – 12.9 %
Tannin	57.3 – 59.1 %
Catechin	14.2 – 17.2 %
Insoluble matter	3.6 – 4.2 %
Non taneris	24.4 – 26.5 %
Ash	1.4 – 1.6 %

What is betel leaf?

The betel leaf contains chlorophyll, small amount of starch, tannin, some volatile oil, chavicol etc. Lime is calcium hydroxide. Catechu is made of tannin and polyphenols. The supari can give rise to carcinogens called, nitrosomines. These are formed in oral cavity due to bacterial action.Chlorophyll in betel leaf is known to have antimutagenic effect. So one should chew betel leaf in combination with betel nut than betel nut alone.

What are the consequences of chewing betel leafs / Pan Masala?

Arecoline of betel nut causes damage to genetic material of mammalion cells. Catechu has also the property of producing harmful effect on cell.

Chewing habit with or without tobacco produces white patches known as leukoplakia. Such oral lesions can progress to cancerous stage. Oral cancer was described in 'Sushruta Samahita' written in Sanskrit around 6 BC.

What about 'Thali type' of food?

It comprises – rice – roti – dal vegetable curd based preparation followed by liberal serving of seasonal fruits. It becomes a complete food supplying most of required nutrients.

Why junk foods are considered inferior to a planned food?

Quite often these fast foods are seen to have a limited nutritive value. They usually have excessive calories, saturated fats, high cholesterol, sugar and salt and very less micronutrient content. Consumption of such foods may be allowed only on occasion.

Should feeding time be a family event?

Yes, It serves very important social and cultural function. Let the daily meeting at the dinning table be a social event in family

Most often, it is the only time when effective interpersonal communication takes place between the family members. It gives an opportunity for elders to monitor the eating and socialising habits of their children.

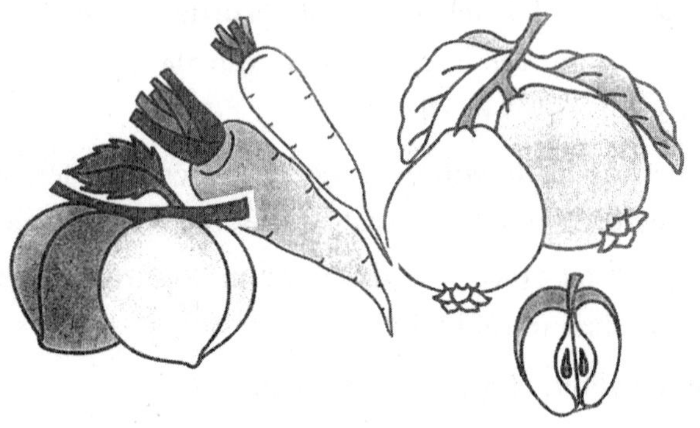

Common Myths About Food

Consumption of raw vegetables is better than cooked one?

Sometimes yes. Diet of raw vegetables and fruits, sprouted seeds nuts/ grains are very rich in vitamin C. E and other oxidants and fiber. This diet reduces certain toxic substances in colon.

But on the contrary some people will find cooked food easier to chew and digest. Cooking makes it easier to absorb some anti oxidants. For example you will get 33% more beta carotene from cooked food. Cooking also increases absorption of lycopene from tomatoes. Broccoli, cauliflowers and cabbage are hard to digest raw. A cooking helps enormously.

Nuts / Seeds are purely fattening?

Three quarters of calories in nuts and seeds come from fats. But nuts and seeds are loaded with antioxidants and other protective substances too. They provide valuable plant protein and fiber. Bulk of fat is a healthy combination of monosaturated and polyunsaturated fats, which help us, absorb and use protective substances.

Taking glass of water with meal is unhealthy?

Food must be chewed thoroughly so that it can be mixed with saliva, which helps in digestion. A glass of water is helpful if it does not take the place of process of mastication.. Taking glass of water before meal will fill your stomach partly so if your dieting it may help but it will dilute gastric juices too hampering digestion.

Late night heavy meal cause weight gain?

Actually time when food is eaten has little impact on weight.

What actually matters is total calorie and fat content. If calories are spread all over the day may promote higher BMR.

But if food is taken at 8'o clock it will be digested partly before going to bed and will have a good sleep.

Only fats are fattening?

No, in excess both protein and carbohydrate can cause excess kilocarie and lead to weight gain.

Pure ghee is most harmful. Vegetable ghee is better?

It is true that pure ghee contains saturated fats more than vegetable ghee. But omega .3 fatty acid content help build cells membrane and support the immune system. They compete with bad cholesterol.

Fat and cholesterol are same?

Fats are similar to carbohydrate that they are composed of carbon, hydrogen and O_2. However they differ in that they contain a greater concentration of carbon leading to higher energy. Saturated fats contain higher hydrogen. If saturated fatty acid predominate the fat is called saturated fat and if unsaturated fatty acid predominate fat is called unsaturated. Lipid is a general term that includes all types of fats. Cholesterol is a fat related compound containing no calories. It is found only in animal fats.

Butter and eggs are rich source of calcium?

No, butter comes from milk fat and does not contain significant amount of calcium. Eggs also don't have significant amount of calcium.

Cured and smoked meat is better?

Nitrates use in cured meats form carcinogen substances in human body. Beckon, sausages, smoked ham have been linked with pancreatic cancer.

Barbecued meat and grilled meat is better?

Barbecued fish contains potent carcinogens. These compounds known as heterocyclic animals enter cells where they damage DNA and start cancer process. Higher the temperature and longer the cooking process, the more chances of forming of carcinogens.

Fat from grilled meat, fish or chickens falling on the flames of barbecue form polycyclic aromatic hydrocarbons. These carcinogens arise from intense heat of a boiler or barbecue and are deposited on surface of meat, chicken. PAHS are related to cancer causing substances in tobacco smoke. They damage DNA starting.

Consuming more of vitamin B complex will give extra strength and protection in body?

No, none of the vitamins contain any calories. Otherwise also water soluble vitamins cannot be retained in body. Excess vitamin is thrown out of body.

Non-vegetarian food gives more strength?

It is wrong. Elephant, horse, genda are all vegetarians. It you combine different vegetarian foods, it become more nutritious.

Skimmed milk is less nutritive?

No, in skimmed milk only fat content is reduced. For heart patient and to reduce weight skimmed milk will prove better.

Consumption of lot of mangoes will result in boils?

Only poor personal hygiene results in boils and not consumption of lot of mangoes.

Does certain foods give more desire for sex?

No, previously it was thought that onions, garlick and non-vegetarian food is 'Tamsi food' or Hot food giving more desire of sex, hence widows, sadhus were not allowed to eat these. But scientifically there is nothing like that. Healthy body gives more pleasure in sex.

ALCOHOL

25% of alcohol is rapidly absorbed from stomach when it is empty. Rest of alcohol is absorbed with in 2 to 6 hours. With in 5 minutes it appears in blood. It traverses freely through placenta to gain access to fetal circulation. It gives 7 calories per gram but does not furnish vitamins or minerals. As regards sex, it gives a desire but takes away the performance.

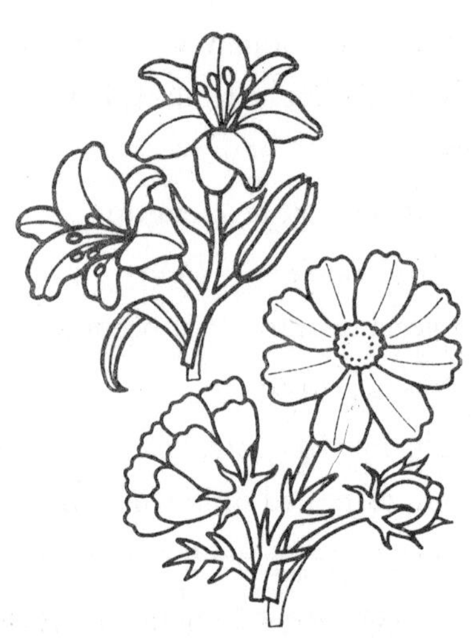

Food & Your Sun Signs

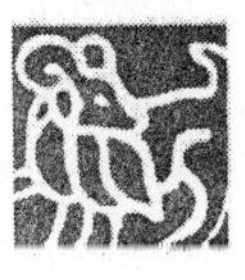

ARIES

Being hot-tempered and straightforward they lack tact. It is best for them to avoid spicy food. They should opt for salads. Simple, vegetarian foods will calm down your volatile moods

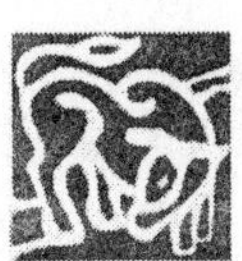

TAURUS

Such person may avoid red coloured food. Red coloured food includes chillies, watermelons, red meats etc. Cool green leafy vegetables, cucumbers, cabbage, paneer soothing to eyes will suit.

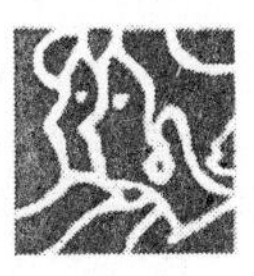

GEMINI

Gemini's are versatile and not boring they have contradictory tastes for foods. They are not choosy as regards food is concerned. They should control their appetite otherwise may become obese which may lead to hypertension and diabetes.

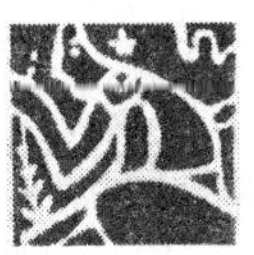

VIRGO

These are fussy about their food. They want exactly as they have asked and need. Extremely quality conscious hence it will better if they cook their own food. They don't enjoy food cooked by servants and becomes critical.

CANCER

These are serious and emotional. These have passion for food and enjoy cooking as well as eating tasty food. They like that other should appreciate food cooked by them. Such females do like to waste food. Their mood swings as well as food choice.

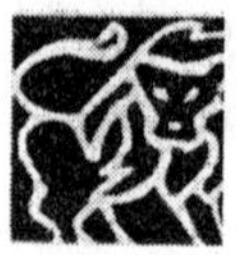

LEO

They enjoy rich and delicious food like lions. Such ladies start secreting saliva as soon as they see food of choice. They just cannot resist. One can approach them through food. Rich fatty food may make them lazy.

LIBRA

These are peace loving and good natured. Their artistic natures like food to be served & prepared in creative way. They love eating but maintain their body figure. They should eat lot of fruits.

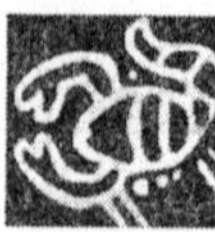

SCORPIO

Being beautiful like good food served in an attractive way. Such female are very fond of ice creams and sweets.

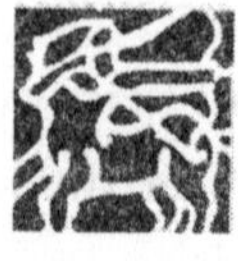

SAGITTARIUS

Cheerful, restless and warm lady. Such female enjoy food they eat full meal and don't believe on dieting. They spend money and appreciate food.

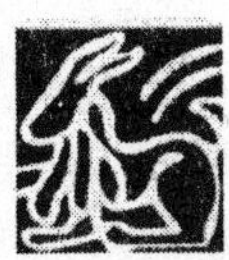

CAPRICORN

These are serious and ambitious. Mostly in India these are vegetarian. These are fond of salad and fruits. They like dairy products.

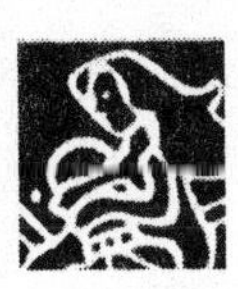

AQUARIUS

Such ladies are honest and friendly. Being analytical while eating such females go on analyzing how such dish would have been prepared. These want to know recipes of their choice food.

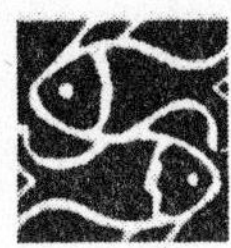

PISCES

Such girls are lovers of music, art and good food. Such ladies are good host in arranging parties and serving food willingly.

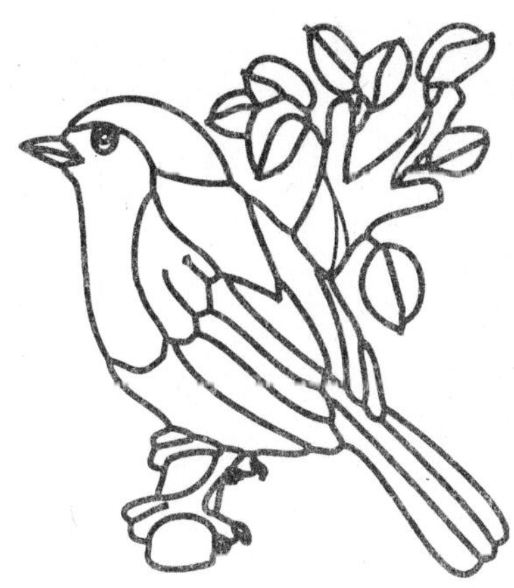

Special Diets in Specific Diseases

1. PEPTIC ULCER

The patient of peptic ulcer should avoid :

- Excessively sour, salty or spicy foods.
- Coarse food such as raw vegetables, fruits with seeds and skin.
- Excessively hot drink/food.
- Smoking, alcoholic beverage and aspirin should usually be avoided.
- Meat should consist of small servings. Try to eat about the same amount at each meal.
- Peptic ulcer is one disease where proper dietary management is equally or more rewarding than pure drug therapy.

Proteins

Nomal protein requirement of 1 gm/kg body weight, i.e. about 60 gm should be given. Milk proteins will not irritate gastric mucosa. Meat soup increases acidity.

Fats

Fat like butter, ghee, cheese and cream are helpful whereas fats of fried food articles are difficult to digest and may increase the symptoms.

Calories

Sufficient calories are to be given and vitamin 'C' may be helpful in healing the ulcer.Lenhart's Diet (After bleeding)

Ist day	2 eggs+ 200 ml of milk
2nd day	3 eggs + 300 ml of milk
Leube's Diet	
Breakfast	One piece bread (50 gm)
Pre lunch	300 ml of milk
Lunch	Mashed potato (50 gm)
	Toasted bread (50 gm)
	Butter (20 gm)
Evening	300 ml of milk
	Biscuit (50 gm)
	Butter (20 gm)
Night	300 ml of milk
Diet Sheet	
Early morning	Milk 1 cup + teaspoonful of sugar.
Breakfast	Bread-2 slices with 10 gm of butter.
	Milk one cup + One Tsf (tea spoon full sugar)
Lunch	Fulka-3 small soft with ghee. Rice one Medium bowl, well cooked dal ¾ bowl, Vegetable ¾ bowl (No Tadka of zeera, etc.)
4 P.M.	Milk 300 ml
6 P.M	Suji porridge

	Suji 20 gm
	Milk 1 cup sugar 2 Tsf
Dinner	Fulka-3 small
	Rice – 1 medium bowl, well cooked
	Dal ¾ bowl, soft bland vegetable ¾ bowl.
Bed time	Time – 1 cup + 1 tsf sugar

Diet will provide 2300 calories and 65 gm of proteins.

2. DIABETES MELLITUS

The following food articles should be avoided.

- Sweet drinks and carbonated drinks.
- Dried and canned fruits.
- Cakes, pastries, cream, and alcoholic drinks.
- Sugar, potatoes.

Diabetes primarily concerns the utilization of carbohydrates in the diet. Insulin which is manufactured in the pancreas is required mainly to convert glucose circulating the blood into glycogen in which form it is stored in the muscles of the body. If insulin is insufficient glucose will build up in the blood and urine.

A diabetic should know how to adjust his diet in order to keep his urine free of sugar.

Carbohydrate

Less than 250 gm should be consumed. But drastic reduction of carbohydrate is forbidden as it might result in excessive metabolism of fat resulting in ketoacidosis.

Calories

Total calories should be adequate for the growing children and underweight persons. For the obsess patients it is necessary to reduce calories. They should consume more of green leafy vegetables which are filling in capacity, low in calorific value and contain less than 3% carbodydrate.

Proteins

1gm/Kg of body weight; cheese is a good source of protein.

Low consumption of fats will keep the cholesterol level low. High doses of B complex vitamin will avoid the development of diabetic neuritis.

Of the minerals potassium helps in release of Insulin from pancreas.Sweetening Agents

There are two chief sweetening agents. One is saccharine in liquid, tablet or granule form. But now a days tab. 'equal' is used.

Saccharine is a coal tar derivative 300 to 500 times sweeter than glucose and does not have any calorific value; of the sugars fructose is the sweetest (173) then sucrose (100), glucose (74) and lactose (60). Sugar free can be used by those obese diabetics who have a craving for sweets. One tables provides only 0.4 calorie which is sufficient to sweeten one cup of tea.

Sorbitol is hydrogenated glucose and is converted into fructose in the body and hence does not cause glycosuria. Tonics of diabetics contain sorbitol.

Diet Sheet

Bed tea	Coffee/ Tea 1 cup

Breakfast	Tea 1 cup 2 toasts with little butter
Lunch	Fulka 2 (two) Rice 1 medium bowl, Dal 3/4th medium bowl. Leafy vegetables 1 bowl, oil for cooking – 1 ½ Tsf.
After-noon	Light tea without sugar
Evening	Fruit one
Dinner	Fulka 2 small, Rice 1 medium bowl or 2 more Fulka, Dal ¾ medium bowl, salad, other Vegetables – 1 medium bowl.
Bedtime	Glass toned milk without sugar.

Approximate calories 1500

Carbohydrate below 230 gm.

3. INFECTIVE HEPATITIS

Proteins

Excessive intake of protein is harmful because of protein break down products may accumulate leading to coma. With mild hepatitis 60 to 80 gm of proteins are permitted.

Fats

May be limited upto 30 gm daily.

Carbodhydrates

Large quantities of oral carbohydrates are given because :

(i) They constitute the major source of calories.

(ii) They minimize the endogenous protein breakdown.

If vomiting / nausea persists intravenous glucose should be given.

For mild jaundice 2000 calories and in severe jaundice 1600 to 2000 calories are recommended.

Vitamin B complex and vitamin 'C' are helpful. Sufficient quantities of sodium chloride and potassium chloride to have electrolyte balance may be consumed.

Diet Sheet

Early morning	Light tea 1 cup with 10 gm sugar
Breakfast	Fruit juice 150 ml + 15 gm sugar Jam 2 tablespoon
10 A.M.	Sugar cane juice 1 glass
Lunch	Rice 2 medium bowl, Thin Dal ½ medium Bowl, butter milk 1 cup + sugar.
4 P.M.	Light tea + 2 Tsf sugar, Banana 1 medium size.
Dinner	Fulka 2 medium size, mixed fruits 250 gm. Well cooked vegetable 1 bowl.

Diet will provide about 2000 calories and 35 gm fat.

4. CHOLECYSTITIS

Food to be avoided are

- Pastries, cheese, fried potato chips.
- Fatty meat, fried eggs
- Cabbage, cauliflower, cucumber, peas and beans
- Nuts, pop corn and dry fruits
- Pickles, condiments and spices.

Proteins

1 gm / kg body weight is permitted, very high protein intake may increase biliary cholesterol.

Fats

Restricted fat diet.

Calories

Minimum carbohydrates to maintain the calories. High carbohydrates will increase the biliary cholesterol.

Fat soluble vitamins may be given.

Diet Sheet

Early morning	Light tea 1 cup with sugar
Breakfast	Toned milk without sugar, Toast 2 with Little jam
Lunch	Rice 1 medium bowl, Fulka 4 small think,
	Thin dal 3/4 th medium bowl, Thin butter milk

	Egg one, Cooked French beans and carrots,
	Oil or cooking 1 ½ spoon
4 P.M.	Light tea 1 cup with 1 tsf sugar
	Biscuits 3 to 4
Dinner	Fulka 4 small, Cooked mixed vegetable 1 bowl, Dal 3/4th bowl, Orange – 1
Bed time	Milk 1 cup without sugar and cream

Diet will provide about 1500 calories, 30 gm fat and 50 gm proteins.

5. ISCHAEMIC HEART DISEASE

Proteins

1 gm / kg of body weight in normal weight patient.

Fats

Saturated fats are to be avoided such as :

Animal fats-beef, meat, pork

Fats procured from dairy products such as cream, butter, ghee.

Hydrogenated vegetables oils.

Unsaturated fats such as Kardi oil, sunflower oil etc. can be used.

Carbohydrates

These are responsible for endogenous synthesis of cholesterol triglycerides. Reduction in sugar intake decreases serum triglycerides.

Calories

Reduction of calories will reduce the weight.

Vitamin 'C' is required for capillary stability. Nicotinic acid reduces lipids in blood, hence both are useful.

Adequate potassium and calcium in blood are required to prevent arrhythmias. Salt restriction is necessary in hypertension of heart failure.

Smoking is hazardous as it produces myocardial oxygen deficiency, increases beta and prebeta lipoproteins and enhances atherosclerosis.

Diet Sheet

Bed tea	Light tea without sugar
Breakfast	Milk one cup without sugar or cream.
Lunch	Fulka 4 small size without ghee.
	Rice one medium bowl, Salad.
	Cooked vegetables 3/4th bowls.
	Oil for cooking 1 ½ Tsf.
4 P.M.	Light tea without sugar and milk
	Sweat lime and papaya.
	Fulka 2 medium size
	Pulses 3/4th medium bowl.
	Salad
	Curd ¾ the medium bowl.
Dinner	Oil for cooking 1 ½ Tsf.
	Cooked vegetables 3/4 th medium bowl.

Diet provides about 1600 calories, 35 gm fats.

5. HYPERTENSION

- Pickles, pastries, salted biscuits, eggs, tinned foods should be avoided.
- Drugs which retain sodium as aspirin, phenylbutazone, corticosteroid should be avoided.
- Extra salt and baking powder should be avoided.

Protein

In milk hypertension 50 to 60 gms of proteins are sufficient. In severe hypertension 40 gm of proteins should be the limit.

Fats

40 to 50 gm of fats are permitted. High intake will cause atherosclerosis, which can cause and aggravate hypertension.

Carbohydrates

It should be the major part to provide calories.

Calories

In obese person low calories will help.

Sodium must be restricted in majority of the hypertensives because sodium has a water retaining property which aggravates the hypertension.

In some cases of low rennin hypertension salt restrictions may be harmful as it may perpetuate the vicious circle of hypertension.

6. ACUTE GLUMERULONEPHRITIS

During severe oliguria, pulses, vegetable soups, pickles, meat and eggs are to be excluded.

Fluid intake should be equal to 500 ml more than the previous day's urine output.

Protein

In severe oliguria protein in take is to be restricted. When urine output is 500 to 800 ml protein intake of 0.5 gm – 0.75 gm per kg of body weight is allowed. If urine output is normal then there is no need of putting protein restriction.

Fats

About 40 to 55 gm is usual because its excretion does not depend on kidney function.

Calories

No restriction.

Vitamins and carbohydrates are to be supplied in normal quantity.

Sodium restriction is necessary so long there is oedema, oliguria or hypertension. Potassium is also restricted in oliguria (green leafy vegetables)

Diet Sheet

Bed tea	Tea 1 cup with 2 Tsf sugar
Breakfast	Milk (150 gm) + Tsf sugar, Bread 2 slices
	With 10 gm of butter
Lunch	Rice 1 ½ medium bowl, Fulka 2 small size,

	Vegetable 3/4th medium bowl.
	Curd 3/4th medium bowl.
Evening tea	Tea 1 cup with 2 Tsf sugar a few potatoes chips.
Dinner	Rice 1 ½ bowl, Fulka 2 , Dal 1 bowl, Vegetable 3/4th bowl. Curd 3/4th bowl.
Bed time	1 cup milk with 1 Tsf sugar

Diet provides about 2100 calories, 50 gm proteins.

7. NEPHROTIC SYNDROME

Following foods may be restricted.

Sodium rich butter, salted biscuits, preserved fish, papad and pickles.

High protein diet 2 to 3 gm/ kg body weight per day is advised as there is massive loss of protein in urine. Ground nut, soya bean, skimmed milk can be frequently used. They can be added to wheat flour. Casilan contains 99% protein and only 0.1 % sodium. Carbohydrates, calories and vitamins requirement remain the same as that of normal man.

When oedema subsides sodium restriction is not necessary.

Diet Sheet

Bed Tea	Light tea with 2 Tsf sugar + 50 ml milk.
Breakfast	Milk one glass with 2 tsf sugar
	Bread 2 slices with 10 gm butter,
	Egg 1 fried or omelette

Lunch	Chapaties 2 medium size
	Rice 1 medium bowl, Dal 1 medium bowl
	Curd 1 medium bowl.
Evening	Roasted ground nut 30 gm, chana 30 gm,
	Milk one glass + 2 Tsf protinex
Dinner	Chapati 3 with ghee, Matar paneer 3 4th bowl or
	Egg 2 as egg curry etc., Dal 3/4th bowl
	Sweet dish 100 gm
Bed time	Milk one glass + 2 Tsf sugar

Diet provides 2600 calories + 95 gm proteins.

8. RENAL FAILURE

Following foods should be restricted :

- Sodium is restricted if there is hypertension, oedema and oliguria
- Salted biscuits, butter, meat, papad, pickles are not permitted.
- Potassium is restricted.

Proteins

With an established disease 40 gm of proteins are permitted.

Half of it should be first class proteins. Usually protein restriction is advocated when blood urea is above 80 mg% . Protein restriction usually varies from 0.3 to 0.5 gm / kg.

Carbohydrates

They help to reduce endogenous protein breakdown and constitute main source of calories. Protein free preparations are allowed in plenty.

Calories

2000 to 2500 calories per day.

Diet Sheet

Bed tea	Light tea with 1 Tsf sugar
Breakfast	Milk 1 cup with 2 Tsf sugar, Bread toast 2 slices With 10 gm of butter.
Lunch	Fulka 4 or 2 medium bowl of rice, Thin dal 3/4th bowl. Well cooked mixed vegetables 1 bowl, Curd ½ medium bowl.
Evening tea	Light tea+2 Tsf sugar, Potato chips, one apple.
Dinner	Rice+Moong Dal khichdi 3 bowl with a Tsf ghee, Raita-Dahi, 1 medium bowl well cooked vegetable, Ice cream 1 small cup
Bed time	1 cup milk + 1 Tsf sugar

Diet will provide 1800 calories, 40 gm of proteins.

9. UNDER WEIGHT

Following should be encouraged :

- Sweetened fruit juices.
- Milk and its products. Cheese, butter and sweets.
- Bread, jam and jelly
- Dried nuts and fruits
- Meat and eggs

Proteins

1.2 to 1.5 gm / kg or more

Fats

These are encouraged to increase weight. These should not be taken in the beginning of food otherwise they will decrease the appetite. Large quantities may produce diarrhoea, flatulence and gastro intestinal upsets.

Carbohydrates

Potatoes, sweet potatoes, biscuits and sweets should be consumed in good quantity. Banana is a good source of calories.

Calories

Total calories consumed should be more than the required to put on weight.

Green leafy vegetables should be consumed in sufficient quantities because these are not good source of calories but may fill up the stomach. Fluids should not be taken before and during meals. Sufficient vitamins are to be consumed.

Diet sheet

Bed Tea	Light tea 1 cup with sugar 2 Tsf.

Breakfast	Milk one cup with sugar 1 Tsf, Bread 2 slices
	Butter 10 gm, Cheese 25 or one egg
Lunch	Fulka 4 small with ghee, Rice one medium bowl,
	Dal one medium bowl
	Curd 3/4 th bowl + 1 Tsf sugar
Evening	Preparation of 50 gm, groundnut
	Fruit juice 1 glass, Banana 1
Dinner	Fulka 2 small with ghee, Fried rice 2 bowl.
	Curd ½ bowl. Dal fry 3/4th bowl.
	Mixed vegetable 1 bowl, Ice cream / sweet 50 gm.
Bedtime	Milk one glass

Diet provides 2800 calories, 85 gm proteins and 105 gm of fats.

10. CONSTIPATION

Proteins

Normal 1 gm/kg body weight

Fats

Ghee and oils are beneficial and act as lubricant to the bowel and stimulate the bile flow for appropriate digestion.

Carbohydrates

Fruits like banana, figs, cucumber with skin and ladies finger are preferred. Cellulose stimulates peristalsis by forming a bulk and facilitate evacuation.

Yeast which is rich in B complex helps to regulate the bowels.

Liberal fluid intake and warm milk intake at bed time are helpful.

11. DIARRHOEA

Food to be avoided are :-

- Deep fry, spicy articles
- Sweets, dry fruits
- Chutney, pickles
- Salad and cellulose containing food.

Proteins

Protein rich substance like skimmed milk, white of an egg, butter milk are helpful. If diarrhoea is due to milk allergy milk is to be avoided.

Fats

Fats will not be absorbed when there is intestinal hurry. They may aggravate the diarrhoea and are best avoided.

Carbohydrates

Easily digested carbohydrates, soft vegetables not with much of cellulose can be given.

As chronic diarrhoea may result in malnourishment high calories may be provided. Diarrohea may result in loss of fluids and electrolytes. They must be replenished orally or in emergency Intravenously.

Salted biscuits, fruit juices and oral electrolyte solutions will be helpful.

12. FLATULENCE

Food to be avoided are :

- Meat, egg
- Cabbage and cauliflower
- High carbohydrates

Proteins

Protein putrefaction in the gastrointestinal tract is the commonest cause of flatulence.

Fats

Fried fatty food stay long in stomach, delayed emptying makes the patient feel uncomfortable.

Carbohydrates

Sweets, potatoes, turnip are to be avoided.

Calories

Obese patients generally do develop gases, hence low calorie diet will be helpful.

13. FEVER

Fever and rest means staying in bed with little physical activity and therefore little need for calories yet to build up the wasted tissue extra proteins are required, i.e. high protein and low calorie diet is required. Hence 70 gm of proteins and 1800 calories will be sufficient.

Proteins can be in concentrated forms such as egg, curds and milk. Fried foods and foods with high fibres should be avoided. Plenty of fluids and minerals should be consumed.

14. GOUT

Person should avoid following foods because these are rich in purine content.

- Vegetarian food-Beans, peas, cauliflower, pulses, lentils, Spinach, apple, mushrooms.
- Non-Vegetarian food- Liver, kidney, fish, meat proteins about 60 gram are enough preferably of vegetable origin.

Fats are to be restricted because they cause urate retention and obesity.

Carbohydrates should form the main part of the diet specially during attack of gout. Carbohydrates can spare proteins which reduce endogenous protein break down.

Low calorie diet will be helpful.

Increased intake of fluid produces increased urine output which will facilitate excretion of uric acid in urine Alcohol and acute attack.

A few cups of tea and coffee are permitted as they contain methyl purines which are not converted to uric acid.

15. PROTEIN ENERGY MALNUTRITION

Proteins – 20% of total calories should be provided from proteins, i.e. about 3 to 3.5 gm per kg of expected body or about 45 to 55 gm of proteins per day. Sufficient quantity of protein is necessary to prevent or treat protein energy malnutrition. Better quality of protein can be got from milk, skimmed milk and pulses. Soya bean is better source of proteins as well as calories.

Fats – It should provide minimum 15-20% of total calories.

Calories – Daily requirement in children is 90-100 calories per kg of expected body weight. National Institute of Nutrition Hyderabad has formulated a rich mixture as follows

Whole wheat roasted	40 gm	
Bengal gram		16 gm
Ground nut		10 gm
Jaggery		20 gm
Total	86 gm	
Total energy		330 Keal
Protein		11.3 gm

Additional banana, egg will help in maintaining good health.

16. 1000 CALORIES DIET CHART

Vegetarian

Morning	Tea 1 cup with milk 2 Tsf and sugar 1 tea spoonful.
Breakfast	Skimmed milk – 1 cup or tea prepared out ot it.
	Toast-1
Lunch	Vegetable soup 1 cup, Thin dal ¾ bowl
	Vegetable salad – radish, tomato, salad

	Leaves, cucumber etc. with salt and pepper.
	Cooked vegetables – pumpkin, French beans, Brinjals etc. except potato, peas, sweet
	Potatoes, etc. No rice, jam, murubba, sweets meat, dry fruits, nuts, soft drinks
Afternoon	Simple tea
Dinner	Tomato soup 1 cup, Skimmed milk curd ½ bowl cooked vegetables, Chapatis, or 'Bread 1 slice, Thin dal ¾ bowl.

Instead of sugar one can use equal or sucaryl in any quantity.

17. 1000 CALORIES DIET CHART

Non Vegetarian

Morning	Tea 1 cup with milk 5 Tsf, sugar 1 teaspoon.
Breakfast	Egg 1 half boiled poached or scrumbled in Milk
	Toast – 1.
Lunch	Meat soup-1 Cup, Boiled fish or roast
	Mutton-moderate quantity. Vegetable salad/ Radish, tomato, salad leaves, cucumber etc.
	Cooked vegetables, pumpkin, French beans
	Except potato, Chapatis 2 or Bread Slices.
	No Rice, jam

Evening	Tea as of morning
Dinner	Chicken soup-1 cup Chicken roast moderate Quantity, Cooked vegetables, Bread 1 slice.

Food Values

Food values per 100 gm edible portion (ICMR : 1971)

Food	Protein gm	Fat gm	Calcium	Iron gm	Vit'C' mg	Vit'A' mg	Caloties
RICE							
Raw milled	6.8	0.5	10	3.1	0	0	345
Parboiled	6.4	0.4	9	4.0	0	0	346
Flakes	6.6	1.2	20	20.0	0	0	346
Puffed	7.5	0.1	20	6.6	0	0	325
WHEAT							
Whole flour	12.1	1.7	48	11.5	0	29	341
Flour refined	11.0	0.9	23	2.5	0	25	348
Suji	10.4	0.8	16	1.6	0	-	348
Bread white	7.8	0.7	11	1.1	0	0	245
MILLETS							
Bajra	11.6	5.0	42	5.0	0	132	361
Jowar	10.4	1.9	25	5.8	0	47	349
Maize	11.1	3.6	10	2.0	0	90	342
Ragi	7.3	1.3	344	6.4	0	42	328
PULSES DALS							
Bengal gram	20.8	5.6	56	9.1	1	129	372
Black gram	24.0	1.4	154	9.1	0	38	347
Green gram	24.5	1.2	75	8.5	0	49	348
Red gram	22.3	1.7	73	5.8	0	132	335
WHOLE DAL							
Bengal gram	17.1	5.3	202	10.2	3	189	360
Green gram	24.0	1.3	127	7.3	0	92	334
Lentil (masur)	25.0	0.7	69	4.8	0	294	343
Peas dry	19.7	1.1	75	5.1	0	39	315
Rajmah	22.9	1.3	260	5.8	0	-	346
Moth beans	23.6	1.1	202	9.5	0	9	330
Soya bean	43.2	19.5	240	11.5	0	426	432

Food	Protein gm	Fat gm	Calcium	Iron gm	Vit'C' mg	Vit'A' mg	Caloties
NUTS & SEEDS							
Ground nut	25.3	40.1	90	2.8	0	37	567
Til	18.3	43.0	1450	10.5	0	60	563
Poppy seeds	21.7	19	1584	-	-	-	408
Cashew nut	21.2	47	50	5.0	-	-	596
Almond	20.8	59	230	4.5	-	-	655
Dry coconut	6.8	62	40	2.7	7	-	662
MILK AND MILK PRODUCTS							
Milk cow	3.2	4.1	120	0.2	2	174	67
Milk buffalo	4.3	8.8	210	0.2	1	160	117
Milk goat	3.3	4.5	170	0.3	1	182	72
Curd	3.1	4.0	149	0.2	1	102	60
Butter milk	0.8	1.1	30	0.8	-	0	30
Cheese	24.1	25.1	790	2.1	-	-	348
Khoa	14.6	31.2	650	5.8	-	-	421
Whole milk Powder	25.8	26.7	950	0.6	4	1400	496
Skimmed Milk powder	38.0	0.1	1370	1.4	5	0	357
EGG & MEAT							
Egg hen	13.3	13.3	60	2.1	0	600	173
Mutton	18.5	13.3	150	2.5	-	0	194
Goat meat	21.4	3.6	12	-	-	-	118
Chicken	26.0	0.6	25	-	-	-	109
Beef	22.6	2.6	10	0.8	2	0	114
Pork	18.7	4.4	30	2.2	2	0	114
Liver sheep	19.3	7.5	10	6.3	20	0	150
FISH							
Pomfrets	17.0	1.3	200	0.9	-	-	87
Hilsa	21.8	19.4	180	2.1	24	-	273
Prawn fresh	19.1	1.0	323	5.3	-	-	89
Fish fresh	11.2	5.8	240	2.3	-	-	138
Fish dry	5.5	2.7	315	3.5	-	-	255
Crab	8.9	1.1	1370	21.2	-	-	59

Food	Protein gm	Fat gm	Calcium	Iron gm	Vit'C' mg	Vit'A' mg	Caloties
GREEN LEAFY VEGETABLES							
Amranth	4.0	0.5	397	25.5	99	5520	45
Bathua	3.7	0.4	150	4.2	35	1700	30
Cabbage	1.8	0.1	39	0.8	124	1200	27
Colocasia							
Green leaves	3.9	1.5	227	10.0	12	10270	56
Coriander	3.3	0.6	184	18.5	135	6918	44
Drumstick							
Leaves	6.7	1.7	440	7.0	220	6780	92
Methi	4.4	0.9	395	16.5	52	2300	49
Lettuce	2.1	0.3	50	2.4	10	990	21
Radish							
Leaves	3.8	0.4	265	3.6	81	5300	28
Palak	2.0	0.7	73	10.9	28	5580	26
BULBS & TUBERS							
Beet root	1.7	0.1	18	1.0	10	0	43
Carrot	0.9	0.2	80	2.2	3	1890	48
Radish	0.7	0.1	35	0.4	15	0	17
Onion	1.2	0.1	47	0.7	2	0	50
Potato	1.6	0.1	10	0.7	17	0	97
Colocasia	3.0	0.1	40	1.7	0	-	97
Yam	1.2	0.1	50	0.6	0	260	79
OTHER VEGETABLES							
Drumstick	2.5	0.1	30	5.3	120	110	26
Capsicum	1.2	0.3	10	1.0	137	420	24
Kerela	1.6	0.2	20	1.8	88	125	25
Beans French	1.7	0.1	50	1.7	24	130	26
Beans cluster	3.2	0.4	130	4.5	49	200	60
Peas	7.2	0.3	20	1.5	9	80	93

Food	Protein gm	Fat gm	Calcium	Iron gm	Vit'C' mg	Vit'A' mg	Caloties
FRUITS							
Amla	0.5	0.1	50	1.2	600	9	58
Guava	0.9	0.3	10	1.4	212	0	51
Grape	0.7	0.1	20	0.2	31	0	32
Lemon	1.0	0.9	70	2.3	39	0	57
Mosambi	0.8	0.3	40	0.7	50	0	43
Orange	0.7	0.2	26	0.3	30	1104	65
Juice	0.2	0.1	5	0.7	64	15	48
Lichi	1.1	0.2	10	0.7	31	0	61
Melon	0.3	0.2	32	1.4	26	170	17
Papaya	0.6	0.1	17	0.5	57	665	32
Pineapple	0.4	0.1	20	1.2	39	++	46
Sitaphal	1.6	0.4	17	1.5	37	0	104
Strawberry	0.7	0.2	30	1.8	52	15	44
Tomato	0.9	0.2	48	0.4	27	350	20
Apple	0.2	0.5	10	1.0	1	0	59
Bael Fruit	1.8	0.3	85	0.6	3	55	137
Banana	1.2	0.3	17	0.9	7	78	116
Cherries	1.1	0.5	24	1.3	7		64
Figs	1.3	0.2	80	1.0	5	162	37
Jack fruit	1.9	0.1	20	0.5	7	175	88
Mango	0.6	0.4	14	1.3	16	2740	74
Chiku	0.7	0.1	28	2.0	6	95	98

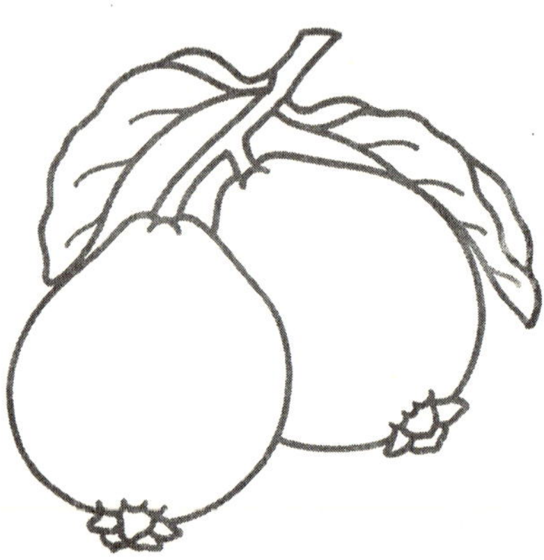

Vitamin Contents of Foods

Food	Carotene (ug)	Thiamine (mg)	Riboflavin (mg)	Niacin (mg)	Folic Acid (mg)	Vitamin 'C' (mg)
Bajra	132	0.33	0.25	2.3	45.5	0
Jowar	47	0.37	0.13	3.1	20.0	0
Maize, dry	90	0.42	0.10	1.8	20.0	0
Maize, tender	32	0.11	0.17	0.6	-	6
Rice, parboiled	-	0.27	0.12	1.0		0
Rice, raw (milled)	0	0.06	0.06	3.9	-	77
Samai	0	0.30	0.09	3.2	9.0	
Wheat flour	29	0.49	0.17	5.5	36.6	-
PULSES						
Bengal gram	189	0.30	0.15	2.9	186.0	3
Bengal gram dal	129	0.48	0.18	2.4	147.5	1
Black gram	38	0.42	0.20	2.0	132.0	0
Green gram	94	0.47	0.27	2.1	-	0
Horee gram	71	0.42	0.20	1.5	-	1
Math beans	9	0.45	0.09	1.5	-	2
Peas	83	0.25	0.01	0.8	-	9
Red gram dal	469	0.32	0.33	3.0	-	25
Soya bean	426	0.73	0.39	3.2	103	0
LEAFY VEGETABLES						
Amaranth	5400	0.21	0.09	1.2	-	169
Cabbage	120	0.06	0.09	0.4	-	72
Carrot leaves	5700	0.04	0.37	2.1	-	79
Colocasia leaves	12000	0.06	0.45	1.9	-	63
Fenugreek	2340	0.04	0.31	0.8	-	220
Lettuce	990	0.09	0.13	0.50	-	10
Curry leaves	7560	0.08	.21	2.3	93.9	4
Mustard leaves	2622	0.03	-	-	-	33
Radish leave	5295	0.18	0.47	0.8	-	81
Spinach	5580	0.03	0.03	0.26	123	28
Turnip green	9396	0.31	0.57	5.4	180	

Food	Carotene (ug)	Thiamine (mg)	Riboflavin (mg)	Niacin (mg)	Folic Acid	Vitamin 'C' (mg)
ROOTS AND TUBERS						
Beetroot	0	0.04	0.09	0.4	-	1
Carrot	1890	0.04	0.02	0.6	15.0	3
Colocasia	24	0.09	0.03	0.4	-	10
Onion	0	0.08	0.01	0.4	6	11
Potato	24	0.10	0.01	1.2	0	16
Radish	4	0.02	0.03	1.4	-	21
Sweet Potato	3	0.06	0.03	0.7	-	24
Tapico	-	0.05	0.10	0.3	-	25
Turnip	0	0.04	0.04	0.5	-	43
Yarn	260	0.06	0.07	0.7	-	0
OTHER VEGETABLES						
Bitter gourd	123	0.07	0.09	0.5	-	88
Brinjal	74	0.04	0.11	0.9	34.0	12
Broad beans	9	0.08	-	0.8	-	12
Cauliflower	30	0.04	0.11	0.9	34	52
Cucumber	0	0.03	0	0.2	14.7	7
Gaint Chillies	427	0.55	0.05	0.1	137	-
Ladies finger	52	0.07	0.10	0.6	105	13
Mango green	90	0.04	0.01	0.2	-	3
Papaya green	0	0.01	0.01	0.1	-	12
Pumpkin	50	0.06	0.04	0.5	13.1	2
Tomato	192	0.07	0.01	0.4	-	31
Tinda	13	0.08	0.08	0.5	-	12
NUTS & OIL SEEDS						
Almond	[illegible]	0.24	0.57	4.4	-	0
Cashew Nut	[illegible]	0.63	0.19	1.2	-	0
Coconut dry	0	0.08	0.01	3.0	16.5	7
Groundnut	37	0.90	0.13	19.9	20.0	224
Pista	144	0.67	0.28	2.3	-	-
Walnut	6	0.45	0.40	1.0	-	0
Gingelly seed	60	1.01	0.34	4.4	134	0
Linseed	30	0.23	0.07	1.0	-	0

Food	Carotene (ug)	Thiamine (mg)	Riboflavin (mg)	Niacin (mg)	Folic Acid	Vitamin 'C' (mg)
SPICES						
Chillies, dry	345	0.93	0.43	9.5	-	50
FRUITS						
Amla	9	0.03	0.01	0.2	-	600
Apricot	2160	0.04	0.13	0.6	-	6
Bael fruit	55	0.13	0.03	1.1	-	8
DATES, DRIED	26	0.01	0.02	0.9	-	3
Figs	162	0.06	0.05	0.6	-	5
Grapes	-	0.12	0.02	0.3	-	
Guava	0	0.03	0.03	0.4	-	212
Jack fruit	175	0.03	0.03	0.3	-	7
Lemon	0	0.02	0.01	0.1	-	63
Mango ripe	2743	0.08	0.09	0.9		16
Orange juice	15	0.06	0.02	0.4	-	64
Papaya	666	0.04	0.25	0.2		4
Pears	28	0.06	0.03	0.2	-	0
Pulm	166	0.04	0.1	0.3	-	5
Strawberry	18	0.03	0.02	0.2	-	52
Tomato	351	0.12	0.06	-	-	
Pineapple	18	0.20	0.12	0.1	-	39
FISHES AND SEA FOODS						
Bhanger	-	-	-	1.8	-	-
Crab muscle	780	-	-	3.1	-	-
Koi	-	-	-	0.5	-	-
Lata	-	-	-	0.8	-	-
Mrigal	-	-	-	0.7	16.7	-
Prawn	0	0.01	0.10	4.8	-	-
Rohu	0.05	0.07	0.7	22		
Shrimp	-	-	-	-	18.6	-

Food	Carotene (ug)	Thiamine (mg)	Riboflavin (mg)	Niacin (mg)	Folic Acid	Vitamin 'C' (mg)
OTHER ANIMAL PRODUCTS						
Beef	345	0.93	0.43	9.5	-	50
Buffalo meat				7.8		
Egg, hen	600	0.10	0.40	0.1	80	-
Goat meat				4.5		
Liver, goat				176.2		
Liver, sheep	-	0.36	1.70	17.6	188.0	20
Mutton		0.18	0.14	6.8	5.8	-
Pork		0.54	0.09	2.8	-	2
MILK AND MILK PRODUCTS						
Milk, buffalo	160	0.04	0.10	0.1	5.6	1
Milk, cow	174	0.05	0.19	0.1	8.5	2
Milk, human	137	0.02	0.02	1.3	3	
Chenna	366	0.07	0.02	-	-	3
Cheese	273	-	-			
Butter	3200	-	-	-		
Ghee,cow milk	200	-	-			
Ghee, buffalo milk	900	-	-			

Mineral Contents of Foods

Food	Magnesium	Sodium	Potassium	Manganese	Zinc
Maize	139	10.9	307	0.48	2.8
Ric, parboiled	61	-	-	0.66	1.33
Wheat,whole	138	17.1	284	2.29	2.7
Bengal gram	119	7.3	808	1.21	6.1
Black gram dal	130	39.8	800	0.96	3.0
Peas, green	34	7.8	79		
Rajmah	184			4.5	
Soyabean	238			2.35	4.4
Cabbage	31			0.18	0.30
Radish leaves	22			0.01	0.08
Spinach	64	58.4	181	0.56	0.30
Onion	16	4.0	127	0.18	0.41
Potato	30	11.0	247	0.13	0.53
Radish white	-	33.0	138	-	-
Bitter gourd	36	17.8	152	0.88	0.46
Cauliflower	18	53.0	138	0.10	0.10
Brinjal	15	3.0	200	0.13	0.22
Cucunber	14	10,2	50	0.14	0.23
Ladies finger	53	6.9	10.3	-	0.42
Mango, green	16	43.0	83	0.07	0.07
Pumpkin	38	5.6	139	0.05	0.26
Tinda	14	35.0	24	0.12	-
Tomato	15	45.8	114	0.19	-
Almond	373	-	-	1.88	3.57
Cashewnut	349	-	-	1.42	5.99
Groundnut	-	-	-	.10	12.20
Walnut	302	-	-	2.32	
Garlic, dry	71	-	-	0.86	1.83
Amla fruit	-	5.6	225	-	-
Apple	7	28.0	75	0.14	0.06
Banana, ripe	41	36.6	88	-	-
Grapes	82	-	-	0.12	0.33
Lemon	19	-	270	0.07	-
Guava	24	5.5	91	0.11	-
Maize	24	-	-	0.14	0.16
Sweet lime			170		
Mango, ripe	270	26.0	205	0.13	0.27
Melon water	13	27.3	160	-	-
Orange	9	4.5	9.3	-	-
Papaya	11	6.0	69	-	-
Pineapple	33	34.7	37	-	-

Food	Magnesium	Sodium	Potassium	Manganese	Zinc
Tomato	-	12.9	146	0.26	0.41
Chingri, dried	-	Copper	1.40	-	-
Helsa	-	52.0	183	-	-
Rohu	13	101.0	288	-	-
Beef muscle	-	52.0	214	-	-
Liver, goat		73.0	160		
Mutton		33.0	270		
Milk, buffalo		19.0	90		
Milk, cow		73.0	140		
Curd		32.0	130